THE NATURAL WAY SERIES

Increasing numbers of people worldwide are falling victim to illnesses which modern medicine, for all its technical advances, seems often powerless to prevent – and sometimes actually causes. To help with these so-called 'diseases of civilization' more and more people are turning to 'natural' medicine for an answer. The *Natural Way* series aims to offer clear, practical and reliable guidance to the safest, gentlest and most effective treatments available – and so to give sufferers and their families the information they need to make their own choices about the most suitable treatments.

Other titles in the Natural Way *series*

THE NATURAL WAY

Asthma

Roy Ridgway

Series medical consultants
Dr Peter Albright MD (USA)
& Dr David Peters MD (UK)

Approved by the
AMERICAN HOLISTIC MEDICAL ASSOCIATION &
BRITISH HOLISTIC MEDICAL ASSOCIATION

E L E M E N T
Shaftesbury, Dorset ● Rockport, Massachusetts
Melbourne, Victoria

© Element Books Limited 1994
Text © Roy Ridgway 1994

First published in the UK in 1994 by
Element Books Limited
Shaftesbury, Dorset SP7 8BP

Published in the USA in 1994 by
Element Books, Inc.
PO Box 830, Rockport, MA 01966

Published in Australia in 1994 by
Element Books
and distributed by
Penguin Books Australia Limited
487 Maroondah Highway, Ringwood, Victoria 3134

Reprinted 1995
Reissued 1998

Cover design by Slatter-Anderson
Designed and typeset by Linda Reed and Joss Nizan
Printed and bound in Great Britain

British Library Cataloguing in Publication
data available

Library of Congress Cataloging in Publication Data
Ridgway, Roy.
The natural way with asthma/Roy Ridgway.
ISBN 1–85230–492-8: $5.95
1. Asthma–Alternative treatment. 2. Naturopathy.
I. Title.
RC591.R53 1994
616.2'3806–dc20   94–25493
CIP

ISBN 1 85230 492 8

Contents

List of Illustrations

For Alex

Acknowledgements

I would like to thank my wife, Dorothea, for her support and cooperation without which I could not have written this important book, my cheerful young friend Timothy for teaching me the reality of the disease of asthma, Dr Donald Lane of the Churchill Hospital, Oxford, for his excellent book *Asthma: the Facts*, Dr David Mrazek, of the Children's National Medical Center, Washington, for his work on the emotional factors in asthma, the UK National Asthma Campaign, the British General, Municipal, Boilermakers and Allied Trade Unions, the UK Chiropractic Advancement Association, Professor John Warner, head of the Child Health Department at Southampton General Hospital, Drs Larry Dossey, John Collins, John Mansfield, David Freed, Duncan Keeley, David Brown and Erika Fromm, director of the Yoga for Health Foundation Howard Kent, aromatherapist Patricia Davis, herbalist Midge Whitelegg, 'natural hygienist' the late Harry Benjamin, and a number of other experts on both sides of the Atlantic for their help in explaining the many gentle ways of dealing with asthma – even though many of them may not be aware they have helped at all because my only contact with them has been through their books and published papers.

Last, but not least, I would like to thank my editor Richard Thomas who has helped me give shape to my research and thoughts and worked hard, with the book's medical advisers Dr David Peters and Dr Peter Albright, to establish a style and standard of excellence for this series as a whole.

Introduction

Asthma has reached epidemic proportions throughout the so-called 'developed world' and the epidemic, particularly among children, is spreading at an alarming pace in almost every industrialized (which means medically-advanced) country, including those in North America, Australasia and Europe.

In February 1994 the largest study of its kind into the disease in Britain found that as many children are dying of asthma now as ten years ago – even though childhood deaths from diseases generally have fallen by nearly a quarter. Most of Britain's more than three million sufferers are children. Childhood asthma accounts for half of all admissions of children to hospital and costs the UK's health service some £107 million a year. Hospital admissions of severe asthma cases have trebled, but among children the figure has risen five-fold. One in seven children now suffers from asthma. In the population as a whole the numbers receiving treatment for asthma have doubled in the past ten years.

The story in America is no different. According to the US National Heart, Lung and Blood Institute, asthma now affects an estimated 12.4 million Americans, nearly double the 1980s figure of 6.8 million. More than four million asthmatics are under 18 years old. The pattern is the same in most developed countries. Even New Zealand, which is not known for the impurity of its air, is affected.

The important fact is that the condition is becoming more common and more severe in spite of campaigns aimed at preventing and controlling asthma through medication. The medication, however, is becoming a problem in itself – as many medical authorities are now beginning to recognize – because of its over-use or misuse.

Writing in the British national newspaper the *Independent on Sunday* in October 1993 journalist Geoffrey Lean pointed out: 'Asthma is the only treatable chronic disease to be advancing, apparently unstoppably, in Western countries, in defiance of an impressive armoury of drugs and treatments.' Asthma prevents people working on over seven million days each year in the UK and estimates for 1990 showed that the cost for asthma in health service charges, social security payments and lost productivity was £750 million.

Though for many sufferers the symptoms are mild, asthma is still a killer. The annual death rate in the UK alone is some 2,000 people – that is, almost one death every four hours. Alarmed at these figures, which are similar in most developed countries, health authorities in New Zealand, Germany and America have now ordered research into the appropriateness and safety of the drugs in common use. Results already coming in show that some asthma drugs – such as inhaled salbutamol or, in the USA, albuterol – not only double a person's sensitivity to an asthma 'trigger' (allergen) such as pollen or dust mites but also set up a strong tolerance, thus reducing its effectiveness.

The problem is: is there still a need for drugs? As most therapists (even natural ones) agree, the sudden withdrawal of drugs can be disastrous for some patients – especially those who have become dependent on them. They are indeed life-saving for some people suffering from severe forms of asthma with chronic inflammation.

Realistically, for these patients the best that can be hoped for is a reduction in the need for drugs, not a complete cure.

This book suggests some more natural ways of dealing with asthma, particulary in the early stages before it gets a grip on a patient, and particularly in the case of children – before they start on what could be a lifetime of drug-taking. In view of the present situation, it seems obvious that there is a need for basic information on what is available by way of natural therapies.

For many doctors and natural therapists the real answer is in the 'holistic' (whole person) approach in which the most appropriate treatment is prescribed for individual patients, whether is natural or conventionally interventionist. More likely, in future, it will be a combination of treatments coupled with plain old common sense and the willingness of the patient to accept responsibility for his or her own health as well as to treat the doctor as an ally and partner rather than as either magician or god.

This book is designed to help asthma sufferers steer clear of the problems, to obtain more effective and, in the main, more natural treatments – and so enable them to live as full, active and trouble-free lives as it is possible for them to do.

Roy Ridgway
Winchester
UK

CHAPTER 1

What is asthma?

How and why it develops, and who it affects

Asthma has experts baffled. We know it is complex and we know it is on the increase but no one has come up with a totally satisfactory definition of what it is. The most that scientists and doctors can really tell us is that it's an extremely complex condition they can recognize but can't precisely define. The nearest they have come so far is to call it 'an inflammation of the airways'.

This 'inflammation of the airways' affects more than half asthma sufferers on most days – so much so, according to a 1991 survey by the UK organization Action Asthma, that it affects their normal daily activities.

Definitions of asthma usually describe symptoms – the dry cough, tightness of the chest, wheezing and breathlessness – not underlying causes like genetic factors, lifestyle, and environmental and psychological problems as well as the immediate triggers. Genetic, lifestyle, environmental and psychological factors are, however, all crucially important – as we shall see. The outcome of a condition such as asthma may even depend on how you approach the illness in the first place: how you react to the initial diagnosis and who you consult afterwards. There are those who believe there may be a critical period in early childhood when asthmatic inflammation becomes established.

For the moment, though, the best most specialists can do is to define it on the basis of its symptoms.

The main asthma symptoms

- *Coughing* – often the first sign of asthma. Sometimes the cough produces mucus that may be white or, if there is an infection, yellow or green.
- *Tight chest* – people with asthma usually describe their chest as feeling tight. Patients will say: 'It's like a heavy weight on my chest', or 'It's like a tight band around my chest.' A New Zealand doctor was even more graphic in his description: 'It's just as if your chest had been blown up with a bike pump and then put into an iron clamp.'
- *Wheezing* – a sort of whistling noise when breathing out.
- *Shortness of breath* – the sensation of not being able to finish each breath before you need another. (Having this symptom does not necessarily mean you have asthma, though. Shortness of breath is common in people when they are under pressure or anxious.) A severe asthma attack can affect sufferers to such an extent they feel they are suffocating to death. One sufferer described it as like 'trying to breathe through a squashed straw while someone sits on your chest'.

How symptoms vary

Perhaps the most distinctive characteristic of asthma is the variability of the symptoms: they usually vary at different times of the day and night and at different seasons of the year. There may be long intervals – months or even years – between attacks or they may be very frequent.

Asthma often happens at night. After a few hours' sleep a sufferer wakes with an irritating dry cough, shortness of breath and a tightness round the chest. Muscles around the neck and shoulders are affected and there is an obvious and audible wheeziness. The wheeziness often occurs in the early hours of the morning. This is known as 'the morning dip'.

The different types of asthma

For many years doctors have seen asthma as being one of two types – one caused by factors outside the body such as the environment, and the other coming from within. These two types are normally called 'extrinsic' (or 'atopic') asthma and 'intrinsic' asthma.

- *Extrinsic* or *atopic* asthma (atopic means 'an inherited allergic tendency') has been seen as characterized by an abnormal sensitivity ('allergy') to food, viral and bacterial infection or inhaled particles such as pollen, dust mite droppings or animal hair. Such environmental factors are known as 'allergens' and allergens are 'triggers' for asthma, in the sense they can trigger asthma off. (The term 'atopic' was introduced in 1923 to describe patients with certain specific conditions that tend to occur together. Asthma and infantile eczema are two such conditions. The unusual sensitivity in these patients is reflected in a special reactivity to the skin. An atopic allergy is what is known as an 'immediate allergy' in the sense a reaction happens within minutes. It is the most common form. The other form is a 'late allergy' in which a reaction happens only after several hours.)
- *Intrinsic asthma* has been seen as a result of something inside you and is believed to be genetic in origin. Specialists who have written about this type of asthma in the past have described a relationship between it and weather conditions at different times of the year. Cold, dry air aggravates the symptoms, causing the airways to narrow. Warm, damp weather can also lead

to difficulty in breathing and some asthmatics experience 'hyperventilation' – literally breathing too much. In most cases hyperventilation is brought on by anxiety and it leads to oxygen starvation.

This distinction between intrinsic and extrinsic asthma is, however, largely out-of-date now. It is really only helpful insofar as it shows some of the ways in which asthma can vary from one patient to another. There are those who do seem to suffer inwardly without its being due to anything outside the body. Yet others are clearly mainly only affected by outside factors such as pollen or animal hair. But asthma defies classification. Many factors may be involved in asthma, both intrinsic and extrinsic – and psychological factors usually interact with physical factors to aggravate the condition. The one thing we can say with absolute certainty, though, is that asthma always affects the body's airways – the lungs and the tubes leading to them – known as the 'respiratory system'.

Inflammation of the airways

Inflammation of the airways is seen as a key factor in asthma. Most medical experts see asthma as nothing else but inflammation of the airways (*see figure 1*). In recent years medical research has concentrated heavily on this side of things. Inflammation results from the release of chemicals produced by cells in the airways. It has even recently been suggested that eradicating these cells may offer the possibility of a cure for asthma.

Recent research by British child health scientists Drs Jill and John Warner of the child health department at Southampton hospital, for example, has found that babies with a high level of activity of these cells – which fail to produce the chemical 'blocking' agent *interferon gamma* – are more susceptible to allergic reactions to dust mites, pollen, animal dander and other triggers. By testing the production of interferon gamma it is possible to establish which triggers affect the baby. Steps can then be taken to protect the baby from exposure to harmful substances.

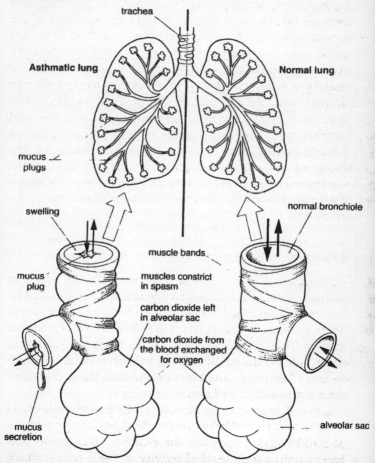

Fig. 1 Asthmatic and normal lungs

This research is now promising enough for an advanced trial to start in late 1994. Researchers are hopeful the outcome of the trial will reduce children's dependence on drugs and medicines – but it is likely to be some years before the tests are available to everyone and meanwhile conventional medicine is concerned mainly at alleviating acute symptoms, controlling chronic symptoms and identifying triggers for asthma to prevent further attacks.

The difference between asthma and bronchitis

Correct diagnosis is the first step in any treatment. How do you know you have asthma and not bronchitis, for example? The symptoms are similar. The word bronchitis means 'inflammation of the bronchi' and wheeziness similar to asthma can be a feature of it. Could 'wheezy bronchitis' be just another name for asthma?

In fact the two illnesses are very different. Bronchitis is not usually accompanied by wheeziness, although it can be. Bronchitis is an infection so, unlike asthma, people with bronchitis normally have a high temperature with 'flu-like symptoms. Unlike asthma, though, people with bronchitis are not fighting for breath like asthmatics, simply wheezing because of the infection. The wheezing is the by-product, not the main condition.

Diagnosing asthma

A thorough examination by your family doctor is an essential first step in any diagnosis of asthma, and probably also a visit to a reliable allergist or clinical ecologist to see which, if any, substances you might be allergic to.

Asthma and allergy tests

There is a link between asthma, hay fever and eczema. Asthma sufferers, and their relatives, often suffer from hay fever and eczema and all these conditions can be triggered off by allergic reactions to the substances listed below.

Sometimes skin tests are used to identify the substances that produce an allergic reaction. Minute amounts of pollen or house dust mite are injected under the skin, and if a patient is allergic to a substance a wheal or rash will form at the site of the injection. Some 96 per cent of asthmatics test positively for at least one of the four main allergens: grass pollen, house-dust mite, pet hair or skin and the common mould *aspergillus fumigatus*.

Diagnosing food allergy is more difficult. Virtually all the tests available are not altogether reliable whether carried out by conventional allergists or those who advocate alternative treatments. The best way to establish a diagnosis is by elimination of suspected foods and, if there is an improvement, conducting a double-blind test. In this test the food is disguised, to avoid bias, so that neither the doctor nor the patient knows what is being tested. A new method using blood samples is being introduced in the US which claims to be much more reliable.

Special note Dietary restrictions should only be carried out with care, and always under the supervision of a properly-qualified dietician or nutritionist. Wrong dieting can be dangerous. Specialists complain that many asthma patients often suffer from the effects of inappropriate and poorly-supervised diets prescribed by someone who doesn't really know what they are doing. For more on special diets see chapter 7.

The main asthma 'triggers'

The following are generally regarded as the main 'triggers' of an asthma attack. They are explained in more detail later:

● *Dust mites* A major cause of an allergic response, these

microscopic creatures thrive in warm places such as carpets or bedclothes in centrally-heated homes. They live by eating the dead flakes of skin from our bodies.

- *Animal danders* A mixture of fur, hair, scale, and urine shed from animals.
- *Pollens* Grass, tree, weed and shrub pollens.
- *Air pollutants* Car exhaust fumes, industrial smog, smoke from coal fires and tobacco smoke. Tobacco smoke, especially, is regarded as a major problem for asthmatics and parents of asthmatic children should keep them away from areas where people smoke, should not smoke in the house and should make sure visitors don't either.
- *Changing weather conditions* A frequent trigger is breathing in dry, dusty air during exercise in hot weather or taking in gulps of cold air in the winter.
- *Exercise* An asthmatic reaction to strenuous exercise can come on quite suddenly or be delayed for five or ten minutes.
- *Food allergies* Dairy products are sometimes a trigger for asthma, as are Chinese food (especially due the extensive use of the preservative *monosodium glutamate*, MSG), highly spiced or salty food such as dry roasted peanuts, packet soups and tinned food (many of which contain MSG). Other triggers include a variety of food colourings, additives and preservatives such as *tartrazine* (E102), a yellow colouring agent added to orange juice products.
- *Hormones* Some women are affected by changes in hormone levels and before periods.
- *Infections* (viruses and bacteria) A viral infection such as a head cold can cause asthma. The asthmatic cough may not go away after a cold. Bacteria do not cause asthma but tend to make the asthma worse. They are caught in the inflamed *bronchi* (see chapter 2) like flies on flypaper.

- *Medicines* Those who develop asthma after puberty may find that they are allergic to aspirin or aspirin-based medicines, non-steroidal anti-inflammatory tablets (for example, Brufen), some blood pressure tablets, and some eye-drops for the eye condition glaucoma.
- *Stress* In stressful situations the body produces hormones such as *adrenalin* and *cortisol* that normally help to improve performance. But when the situation giving rise to the fear and anxiety is purely 'psychological' and does not call for increased physical activity the body is overloaded with hormones it cannot use. This leads to increased heart rate, high blood pressure and other physical damage. It can also trigger an asthma attack.
- *Moulds* Fungi which grow in damp houses, the soil of house-plants, conservatories with moist air and so on can trigger attacks.

The immune system and asthma

Our body's immune system is often compared to an army fighting off invaders. The troops are the anti-bodies that are summoned to attack and destroy any invader, such as a virus, as soon as it enters the body. While the battle continues the temperature is raised and other things happen such as the sweats and rashes many of us get when we have a viral infection like 'flu. The symptoms only subside when the immune system 'army' gains the upper-hand over the invader – as, in most of us, it normally does.

In some people, though, the troops seem to be called out at the slightest excuse. In allergies, for instance, the immune system reacts in what seems like an incorrect way to a substance called an *allergen*. But the reaction may not be incorrect. Though the invading army may have no big guns it may be more deadly than it seems.

Morover they are supported by a fifth column – medication (drugs) – which tricks the defending army into believing that nothing much is wrong.

The seemingly wrong reaction – or rather over-reaction – is called an 'allergic reaction'. In this kind of reaction our bodies produce a special type of antibody known as *immunoglobulin E* (IgE for short). IgE activates special cells called 'mast cells'. Mast cells release a number of chemicals that cause the symptoms of allergy. The best-known of these is *histamine*. It is histamine that is responsible for the spasm and narrowing of the airways in the lungs that lead to an asthma attack.

Problems with new conventional treatment

Recently US health officials, concerned about the rise in asthma, asked doctors to be more aggressive in their use of asthma treatments and in training young people to manage their asthma as early as possible. This advice followed the recognition that inflammation is difficult to control once it has become established. All the treatments the US health authorities recommended were aimed at dealing quickly with acute symptoms, preventing further attacks and controlling chronic symptoms.

When the number of treatments rose as a result of this campaign the health authorities were pleased – until a complication arose. It was pointed out that even though the number of new treatments was rising so also was the number of asthma deaths. And indeed a similar story was emerging in many other countries where an aggressive treatment policy had been adopted.

Fearing that some of the treatments were doing more harm than good the US National Heart, Lung and Blood Institute has now launched a major study to find out the long-term effects of its policy. The institute has recruited nearly a thousand children, girls and boys, aged from five to 12 for its 'Childhood Asthma Management Programme' (CAMP).

CAMP researchers are following the children at eight medical centres in America for at least five years. The aim is to determine the safety and adverse effects of various drug therapies and measure such factors as lung function, frequency of asthma attacks, physical development and quality of life. It also hopes to resolve a medical debate: some doctors recommend giving children medicine every day as a matter of routine – even if they suffer from only occasional mild symptoms. Others believe the children should receive medicine only when they are ill and have symptoms.

Reflecting on the uncertainties of conventional asthma therapies and the puzzles about the asthma epidemic, Dutch asthma expert Dr Ruurd van Rourda – who has already collaborated with American experts in research showing that many children with moderate or severe asthma do not, as many think, altogether outgrow their asthma (see box 'Do children outgrow their asthma?') – said in January 1994: 'Asthma is not as simple as once thought.'

Do children 'grow out of' asthma?

It is generally believed that most children 'grow out of' childhood asthma. But recent research in the Netherlands by Dutch physician Ruurd van Rourda suggests that many children with mild to severe asthma in childhood do not grow out of it. Their asthma does get better in their late teens or early twenties because their airways grow larger but in many cases the underlying problem remains.

Dr Rourda says the reason young adults give up medication is more to do with their becoming used to their symptoms, and so being able to cope without medicine, rather than being 'cured' of asthma. 'Children grow out of their doctors rather than their asthma,' Dr Rourda was quoted in the *New York Times* in January 1994.

In Britain another specialist, Professor Peter Barnes, admitted in October 1993: 'We still know very little about the long-term outcome of asthma and prolonged trials of treatment are needed.'

A better understanding of the disease may lead to better treatment. Research aimed at identifying triggers in early infancy, even before birth, is possibly a step in the right direction. But at the moment the dramatic fact is that conventional treatments are simply not working and natural therapies – which may include preconception care of couples with a history of asthma – may offer the best hope for many sufferers.

But before we look at the details of the various treatments on offer, both conventional and natural, as well as how to avoid asthma and help yourself it is necessary to understand more about the importance of breathing and the lungs, including how they work and why they go wrong.

CHAPTER 2

All about breathing and the lungs

How it works and why it's important

We talk of the 'breath of life' and that is precisely what it is – the air we breathe is essential for life. It is the most essential thing the human body needs. We can live for days without water and weeks without food but only a matter of minutes without air. The most important ingredient in air is *oxygen*. Oxygen is necessary to 'burn' foods to produce energy. This 'burning' process is known as 'aerobic metabolism' (the word 'aerobic' means 'requiring oxygen to live', and 'metabolism' is the word for the chemical processes that take place in the body).

How the body takes in oxygen

Oxygen is taken in and absorbed by the body through the lungs and the bloodstream *(see figure 2)*. Air is breathed into the lungs and oxygen from the air then passes into the bloodstream via millions of tiny little blood-surrounded air sacs in the lungs known as *alveoli*. The 'oxygen-rich' blood is then pumped through the left side of the heart and the arteries to all parts of the body until it reaches the minute blood vessels called 'capillaries' that interweave every piece of human tissue. The tissues absorb the oxygen from the blood, together with other essential nutrients and chemicals, and so fuel the energy processes which give us life.

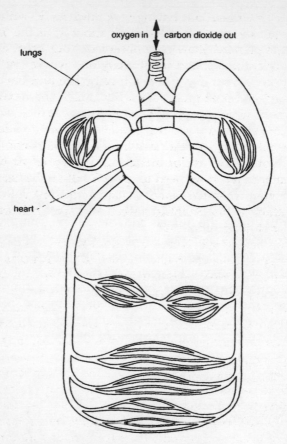

Fig. 2 Breathing and circulatory systems

A waste product of this energy process is *carbon dioxide*. As the tissues absorb oxygen from the bloodstream so they send back carbon dioxide. Carbon dioxide is of no value to the body so it is expelled by being returned to the lungs through the veins and the right side of the heart and back into the air every time we breathe out.

This remarkable exchange process goes on throughout

our lives without our having very much to do with it. It only goes wrong when we think about it, as the writer George Bernard Shaw once observed. Your breathing is mostly automatic and involuntary and works perfectly well on its own if you live a healthy life and have not learned bad breathing habits. But unlike the heart, for example, which works automatically and which we can do little to control, breathing can be both automatic and controlled. Singing and shouting are both examples of our 'voluntary' use of breathing. It may let us down sometimes when we need to speak loudly to be heard or in singing when we cannot sustain a note but voluntary breathing is important in speech and such performing arts as singing and acting.

The British specialist Dr Donald Lane, a consultant physician at the Churchill Hospital in Oxford, has written vividly about this double talent of our breathing system, and particularly the muscles which control it:

'The muscles of breathing are unique amongst the body's musculature. They can be moved at command but also operate automatically. We can fill our lungs full of sea air. We can hold our breath to keep out smoke. We can shout or sing. The use of the muscles of breathing in these ways is akin to the use of arm or leg muscles for writing or walking. But whereas arm and leg muscles remain stationary unless we will them to move, the muscles of breathing do not. They have an involuntary or automatic rhythm of their own. Whether we are dozing in a chair or running for a bus, the muscles of breathing keep up their regular movement. In this respect they are behaving like the muscles of the heart. Heart muscle action is, however, almost wholly automatic and we have very little, if any, voluntary control over it. So the unique nature of the muscles of breathing lies in their dual control, for the most part automatic, but available for voluntary use.'

But how do these muscles work? How in fact do we breathe? Why do some people get asthma and not others? What triggers things off in the first place, and why? To understand the answers to these key questions we need to look closer at the lungs, the mechanics of breathing and at the muscles involved in the breathing process.

The normal lung

When the normal healthy person breathes in, air passes through the nose and mouth into the *trachea* or wind pipe. The trachea divides into two main airways called *bronchi*, and these in turn divide into smaller and yet smaller branches called *bronchioles*. At the end of the bronchioles are, as we have already seen, tiny air sacs called *alveoli* where oxygen is exchanged for carbon dioxide via the bloodstream. This system is known as the 'respiratory tract' and the process of breathing is called 'respiration'.

The whole of the respiratory tract, including the nose, trachea and airways, could be compared to a sort of air-conditioning system whose function it is to convert every sort of air – clean or polluted, hot or cold, humid or dry – into clean, moist air for delivery at body temperature to the aveoli.

The lining of the airways produces mucus for trapping dust particles. The airways also contain millions of microscopically small hairs called *cilia* that all beat in unison a thousand times a minute to sweep the mucus to the top of the trachea where it can be swallowed. Coughing and sneezing have the effect of expelling mucus from the airways.

Two sets of muscles wrap round the airways in a double spiral, like Greek sandal thongs. In a healthy person these muscles open the airways during exercise and close them as a protective mechanism in, for example, a smoky room. The lungs are a natural protection against disease, but they don't work so well when they are weakened by too much industrial or domestic dust and dirt, car exhaust fumes and other irritants.

When you breathe rhythmically and easily your body is supplied with all the oxygen it needs for energy production, and it is able to get rid of all the carbon dioxide from the blood in an efficient way. When this exchange process is functioning as it should you enjoy good health and are able to cope when your body is called upon to make a special effort – as it does, for instance, in cold weather or when running for a bus, or carrying a heavy load of shopping or climbing lots of stairs. For those prone to asthma, exertion of this kind can quickly bring on breathlessness or wheezing.

The asthmatic lung

Everybody's airways narrow and expand according to environmental conditions, but in an asthmatic attack the airways become inflamed and swollen which has the effect of narrowing them. An excess of mucus is formed that clogs the airways and the airway muscles may then go into spasm, causing further narrowing.

That is what happens physically. But there is more to it than this. A major role in the breathing process, and also why some people get asthma and others don't, is played by our emotions. Emotions, as well as being closely associated with breathing, are also crucially linked to the body's autonomic nervous system.

The autonomic nervous system

The autonomic nervous system controls the famous 'fight or flight' response that has been part of the human system since the very earliest days of our evolution when our ancestors had to live on their instincts to survive. The autonomic nervous system actually consists of two opposite but supporting systems known as the 'parasympathetic' and 'sympathetic' nervous systems:

- *The sympathetic nervous system* heightens activities in the body, raising blood pressure and blood sugar levels, quickening the heartbeat, widening the pupils of the eyes and dilating the main airways, and diverting blood from the skin and digestive organs to the muscles and brain.
- *The parasympathetic nervous system* has the opposite effect, slowing heart rate, lowering blood sugar levels, constricting the airways, and transferring blood to the digestive organs.

Today we don't have sabre-toothed tigers to contend with but we do have to deal with teachers, parents, the boss, the bank manager and a host of other equally stressful psychological conditions and situations. Psychological events can influence breathing rhythms by affecting the airways and causing them to contract through the parasympathetic nervous system.

It works like this: between a nerve and a muscle there is a tiny gap. This gap is bridged by a so-called chemical 'messenger' known as a *neurotransmitter*. Different chemicals called *hormones* do the bridging in different parts of the nervous system. For the sympathetic nervous system, for example, the transmitter is the hormone *epinephrine* or *adrenaline* (better known just as 'adrenalin'). For the parasympathetic nervous system it is *acetylcholine*.

The autonomic nerve pathways of the lungs are activated by what is called a 'reflex'. Reflexes are one of the ways in which the body responds to outside influences or 'stimuli'. Reflexes are built-in automatic responses that are not the result of a conscious decision to do something. They just happen. A typical reflex action is dropping a hot plate if it is handed to you. You don't have to think about it. You just drop the plate without conscious thought. Other reflexes control balance, movement, posture – and breathing.

In the case of asthma, the reflex action of the parasympathetic nervous system causes the small airways (*bronchioles*) to contract, resulting in coughing and wheezing. This is called *broncho-spasm*.

Why breathing goes wrong

When you breathe in the diaphragm, which is a dome-shaped sheet of muscle underneath the thorax, is pulled flat. This has the effect of pulling the rib-cage upwards and outwards, causing the lungs to expand and air to be sucked into them (*see figure 3*). The stronger the muscle action the more air enters the lungs.

Breathing function reflects your state of mind. The diaphragm does the work when you are relaxed and your breathing becomes rhythmic and slower and your lungs receive all the oxygen they need. But much of the time many people breathe fairly rapidly and shallowly using mainly the chest muscles and this can upset the delicate balance of oxygen and carbon dioxide in the body. Because breathing goes wrong at times of stress diaphragmatic breathing and relaxation exercises are particularly important for asthmatics.

Haphazard breathing

Mood changes are well known to change our breathing pattern. Much of our breathing is haphazard as a result. We do not notice this because we have become accustomed to breathing in this irregular way. There are those who go so far as to say that, for many of us, our breathing went wrong at the start of our lives: we were born

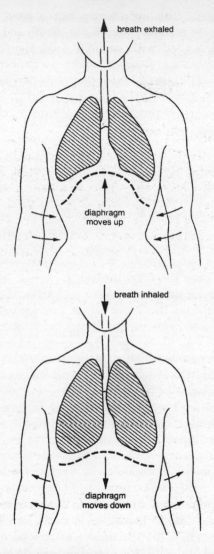

Fig.3 How to breathe properly

under bright lights and thrown into a panic when we were forced to breathe through the mouth and nasal passages still clogged with *amniotic fluid*, the fluid in the mother's womb we 'swim' in before we're born.

Various childbirth pioneers have drawn attention to this. The theory is that the memory of the gigantic struggle to be born and draw our first breath remains in our system as body tensions and feelings of insecurity. 'We learned to breathe in the middle of pain,' as the psychotherapist Leonard Orr has put it. He teaches a form of therapy called 'healing the breath' to overcome precisely this problem.

Why breathing goes wrong in asthma

In asthma the delicate mental, emotional and physical balance that seems to be necessary in so many human functions is upset. It is as if the 'automatic pilot' gets switched off and someone inexperienced takes over the controls. This shows itself in an increased sensitivity to everyday influences and surroundings, or 'stimuli', from car-exhaust fumes and the dust in our centrally-heated homes with their wall-to-wall carpets to the pressures at work and at home. All these things then become potential 'triggers' for an asthma attack.

All aspects of life are nourished and sustained by breathing so anything that interferes with this vital function is interfering with the most fundamental of all requirements for living. We can look at the body as an amazingly complex machine built to perfection, a sensitive machine that will break down if it is not treated with respect. And like all machines, it needs repairing from time to time: it needs the right sort of food to keep the parts functioning efficiently, and it needs to be used regularly and correctly to prevent it from deteriorating.

In this sense there's no doubt – as all practitioners and

therapists agree – that drug medicine and surgery can very often be essential tools in the repair and maintenance of the human machine. But, unlike a piece of engineering, the body is mainly self-sustaining and self-repairing. Factors other than the physical – such as the mind and emotions – are always involved in sickness and health, and breathing is one of the most directly affected: hopes, fears, anxieties and similar emotions have a close and intimate effect on breathing.

Breathing and feeling

So breathing is closely related to feeling, but in most clinical descriptions of asthma the major life events, or even the events of everyday life and their effect on the course of a disease such as asthma, are not mentioned. Yet everything that happens in our lives, from what happens in the home and community to what happens on the world stage, has some bearing on our health – which is why various experts have tried to understand the psychological aspects of asthma.

Asthma is sometimes said to be connected with repressed emotions and so it may be helped by learning to express feelings. Is the asthmatic perhaps someone who tends to feel too much, who is perhaps too sensitive, mentally and emotionally as well as physically, to the world and its woes?

Feeling may be central both to an understanding of asthma and its treatment. Laughing and crying can change the flow of breathing and, in a susceptible individual, trigger an asthmatic attack – as can almost anything that involves too great a change in breathing rhythms such as gasping in horror or holding the breath in suspense.

It's time to take a closer look at these likely causes and triggers.

CHAPTER 3

Causes and risk factors in asthma

How lifestyle and emotions can trigger an attack

The full story about the exact causes of asthma is not yet clear but the following are probably the major 'risk factors', as they are called:

- inherited tendency
- nutritional deficiencies
- viral infection in infancy
- stress
- environmental pollution
- inappropriate exercise.

Inherited tendency

Asthma's link to the genes you inherit from your parents is well known – though experts are unsure about the exact details and how it all fits in with other factors. Professor Peter Barnes, head of thoracic medicine at the National Heart and Lung Institute in London, for example, has said: 'The quest for the single "asthma gene" is unlikely to be rewarding as a complex interplay between many genes and several environmental factors is likely to exist.'

What studies so far have shown, though, is that if neither of your parents has asthma the risk of your being asthmatic is about 15 per cent. If one of your parents has asthma this risk increases to 30 per cent. If both your parents have asthma your risk rises to 60 per cent.

The risk varies from country to country, so environmental influences probably also play a part. 'Allergic asthma' is five times more common in Australia than Britain, for example, and 20 times more common in Britain than China or Hong Kong. Time of birth may also be significant. It is known, for instance, that babies born during the pollen season risk developing hay fever, which in some ways resembles allergic asthma, in later life.

Nutritional deficiencies

Experts in nutrition believe that diseases running through families may be caused not only by inherited characteristics but also, or even entirely, because of shared problems such as poor diet. There is evidence, for example, that poor eating by the pregnant mother is a cause of some birth defects. Babies who don't weigh much when they're born have a higher-than-average risk of developing diabetes and cardiovascular disease later in life. We also know that a poor diet in pregnancy, particularly a diet low in folic acid (one of the many B vitamins), is a cause of some neural tube diseases such as *spina bifida*. Correct nutrition is extremely important in the early stages of the development of the baby in the womb (*embryo*) when nerve cells are forming.

Viral infection in infancy

Babies who catch a viral infection are believed to have a greater chance of developing asthma later in life as a result of having inflamed airways and a weakened immune system at such an early stage.

Stress

One of the most important, if altogether less clear, causes of asthma is stress. The link between emotion and stress is well known but not so the link between stress and asthma.

Trousseau, a famous nineteenth-century French physician who was himself asthmatic, has written of how his worst attack of asthma happened in a grain loft. The air was dusty but on this occasion there was also something else 'in the air'. Trousseau suspected his coachman of dishonesty in measuring some grain and had therefore decided to supervise the operation himself: 'I had a hundred times been exposed to an atmosphere of dust considerably thicker... [This time it] acted on me whilst I was in a peculiar state. My nervous system was shaken from the influence of mental emotion caused by the idea of a theft, however trifling, committed by one of my servants.'

This reaction has actually been put to the test. During a consultation with an asthmatic patient a researcher released a small amount of pollen, normally not enough to cause any wheezing, into the atmosphere. The patient was unaware of this – but when he started discussing some unpleasant aspects of his life with the researcher, which provoked feelings of anger or fear, the wheezing started. It stopped as soon as the subject was dropped.

Dr David Mrazek, chief of psychiatry and behavioural sciences at the Children's National Medical Center in Washington DC, has also found that emotional and non-emotional factors can interact in asthma. The less severe allergic reaction – as in the case of a nervous and suspicious person prone to bouts of bad temper such as Trousseau – may be quite enough to trigger an attack.

No-one has so far been able to predict an attack purely on the grounds of personality, though. Experts who

have studied the connection between disease and personality (known as 'psychosomatic medicine') have not
come up with any specific personality trait in the asthmatic, although the inability to assert themselves is said
to be one characteristic. Asthmatics do not seem to fall
into any one psychological group.

Dr Mrazek has identified characteristics he believes
may be individual responses to stress – but he thinks
these may be due more to an inherited vulnerability than
acquired personality traits. Thus in the person who is
genetically programmed to have a hyperactive nervous
system – in other words, jangly nerves – 'stress and
arousal will send a volley of nerve impulses to the airways,' he says. So in the person already genetically predisposed to asthma this could result in the airways
becoming constricted with a feeling of tightness in the
chest and shortness of breath. This, says Mrazek, seems a
likely way in which stress symptoms could trigger asthmatic attacks in susceptible people.

In a study by Mrazek and colleagues of 150 children
at risk for asthma because they had one asthmatic parent
a strong connection was established between early 'stres-
sors' (stress factors) and the onset of asthma. They found
that when stress situations in the family, such as the
death of a close relative or an unexpected job loss, came
at a greater than average rate in the year before the child
was born the child was more likely to develop wheezing
at two years old. The stresses that occurred before birth
were likely to go on in the months after and the turmoil
in the home would probably have affected the child's
ability to deal with emotions.

Environmental pollution

There are now indications of a new class of asthma-suf-
ferer, one who is not genetically predisposed to the dis-

ease. He or she may be a child of parents who have no history of asthma at all but the child still develops asthma. Living near a main road with heavy traffic, and therefore a high level of air pollution, is one possible suspect that has been identified. Many now believe environmental pollutants are a major reason for the rapid rise of asthma in the West.

They believe this accounts for the fact that although asthma is affecting children in increasing numbers few of them fall into the category of 'old' asthmatics. That is to say, they have not had both eczema and asthma from infancy so they are unlikely to have an inherited 'allergic tendency' towards asthma.

Pollution hits children hardest because their airways are narrower. Children under three breathe in twice as much air as adults for each pound of their body weight. Children are usually very active and exercise more than adults and therefore take in more air and more pollution.

Links between asthma trends and environmental pollution is the subject of research going on at the moment but results so far seem to point the blame at two particular pollutants from car exhausts: ozone and nitrogen dioxide.

- *Ozone*, which is a life-saver in the stratosphere, screening out the harmful ultraviolet rays from the sun, is a killer at ground level. Concentrations of it cause damage to human tissue. Research in the US has linked ozone with lung damage as well as asthma.
- *Nitrogen dioxide* has the same kind of effect and was described in a British government report early in 1993 as giving the 'greatest concern' of all air pollutants. Nitrogen dioxide accumulates in towns and cities because of traffic. Emissions from car exhausts have increased by 73 per cent since 1981, and in 1992 another

British government study reported that 19 million Britons were exposed to pollution that exceeded European Community (EC) guidelines. Studies in Canada, Switzerland and Sweden have also implicated nitrogen dioxide in asthma.

Asthma symptoms are also caused by lead, mercury, cadmium, aluminium and arsenic so any air polluted with these highly poisonous metals – for example, fumes from an industrial plant – is another source of trouble.

International pollution research

Opponents of the 'pollution causes asthma' case say pollution cannot cause asthma even though evidence to that effect is mounting all the time. The present consensus is that if pollution is not a cause of asthma it certainly aggravates it.

In the UK, work at the East Birmingham Hospital has shown that when levels of pollution rise more people are admitted to hospital with asthma attacks. In October 1993, London's famous St Bartholomew's Hospital published research showing that both ozone and nitrogen dioxide damage the lining of the lungs and the tubes we breathe through. Substances that can trigger off asthma get into the lining and damage the tiny hairs (*cilia*) that remove infection from the lungs, so accelerating the inflammation that brings on an attack.

At a meeting in 1993 some 400 top British chest specialists agreed that air pollution made asthmatics worse. Dr Malcolm Green, chairman of the British Lung Foundation, was quoted in the media at the time as saying: 'If pollution is making people with bad asthma worse, and makes those with a little suffer more attacks, it is quite likely that those on the threshold of asthma may be tripped over.'

Smoking
All doctors will warn patients of the dangers of smoking which obviously will further damage the lungs of asth-

matics and aggravate the condition. Symptoms of asthma are twice as common in the children of parents who smoke. A 1993 American study of 199 children showed how inhaling tobacco smoke aggravated asthma. Tobacco exposure was determined by measuring the level of *cortinine* (a derivative of nicotine) in the child's urine. High levels of cortinine was associated with an increase in 'acute exacerbations' of asthma and a deterioration in the way the lungs worked.

Another study carried out in the UK by Dr John Britton at the City General Hospital in Nottingham gave further evidence of the link between mothers who smoke and asthma in their children. 15,000 children born in one week in 1970 were studied for risk factors. Factors such as the age of the mother, social class and income, whether or not the children were breast-fed, and the size of a family were all linked in some way with wheezing.

But the data on smoking proved the most dramatic. Some 30 per cent more children whose mothers smoked showed asthma symptoms by the age of 16 than those of mothers who didn't. Low birth weight was also a risk factor. Fifty per cent of the children in the study who weighed under 3lb 3oz (1.45kg) at birth experienced wheezing illnesses by the age of 16.

Exercise

Almost all asthma sufferers will find that any form of vigorous exercise will bring on asthma symptoms. The asthma starts during exercise but lasts after the exercise ends. Instead of being able to relax afterwards and get his breath back, the sufferer may find that a rapidly worsening fit of wheezing overtakes him.

What happens normally is that the airways widen during exercise and then quickly settle back to their previous state afterwards. With asthmatics the airways

reach their narrowest between about three and five minutes after the end of exercise, remain like that for a
while, and then gradually widen to their pre-exercise
level. The degree of increased narrowing can last for two
or three hours.

Exercise is not all bad, however, and the right sort of
exercise can help rather than hinder the asthmatic. In
chapter 4 we'll look at the positive side of the picture.

How to help yourself

Rules and guidelines for avoiding asthma

The first step in helping yourself is to decide you want to do something to help yourself. There is a lot that can be done to avoid asthma in the first place, and then to prevent it or alleviate the symptoms if you can't avoid it. This chapter is all about taking those avoiding steps, and if you can't avoid everything that might trigger an asthma attack it is important to know what to do to tone down the attack and/or even eliminate it altogether. It is about treating yourself in other words.

Avoiding asthma

Avoiding asthma is mostly a matter of common sense. The British National Asthma Campaign, for example, gives out rules for avoiding an asthma attack based on those below, and similar guidelines are recommended in other countries:

- Avoid cigarette smoke and don't smoke yourself.
- Wrap a scarf round your face on cold days.
- Exercise outside on warmer days (unless pollution levels are high) and inside on cold ones. Always remember that exercise, while generally good for you, can also sometimes cause breathing problems so avoid rushing around.

- Keep tension to a minimum.
- Keep healthy.
- Avoid people with a chest virus if possible.

If the asthma is due to a known allergic reaction, you can take the following action:

- Don't keep warm-blooded pets.
- Check to see if food labels include ingredients that you are allergic to.
- On hot dry days don't spend too much time outdoors.
- In summer avoid long grass and close car windows.
- Remove any mould or fungus in the house quickly.
- Avoid damp.
- Don't keep old clothes.

At work
Conditions to avoid at work are:

- Industrial fumes and dangerous chemicals. Some innocent-looking chemicals in the office may cause problems. Talk to your local Health and Safety Executive office (UK) if you are concerned (*see figure 4*, pp. 38-9).
- People who smoke.
- Too much stress. Learn to balance your workload.

There are many things everybody can do to minimize health risks in the workplace – including observing the health and safety regulations yourself. But you should not hesitate to take the matter up with your local health and safety officer if you are asked to do anything or work in conditions that are likely to cause a risk to your health. In most countries, but especially in European Community countries, the law is on your side. Indeed under EC law your employer must do something about it if there is a risk to health . Dust levels, for example, must be kept low. The control of dangerous dusts usually involves special measures to suppress dust and exhaust

Can air control devices help?

Opinion is divided about whether devices like ionizers and
humidifiers (and de-humidifiers) are helpful for asthmatics.
Some specialists say yes and others no.

Ionizers are devices which neutralize the positive ions in the
air and replace them with healthy negative ions. Ions are
charged particles of carbon dioxide, nitrogen and oxygen.
Negative ions are good for us because the air in places like
the sea or up mountains that we know are good for us is full
of negative ions. The insides of cars, houses and factories,
on the other hand, usually have more positive than negative
ions in the air. Some people claim it is too many positive
ions in the air which can lead to headache and tiredness,
and so having an ionizer can help counteract these symptoms. But ionizers also collect air pollutants like dust and
pollen and so probably benefit asthmatics too.

Humidifiers and *de-humidifiers* are simply devices that either
make the air more moist (humidifier) or less moist (de-
humidifer). Though adding moisture or removing it can obviously help asthma sufferers in situations where the air is
either too dry (such as in most centrally-heated homes with
double-glazing) or too damp (such as in some old or sub-
standard buildings) most specialists regard them as an
unnecessary expense. They say houses where the air is too
dry can be improved by

- regularly opening windows and letting in fresh air from outside
- placing a container of water on or near radiators or
  heaters (a wet towel over a radiator – *but not a heater of
  course* – will work just as well).

Houses where damp is a problem will also benefit from letting in as much fresh air as possible, especially on days
when the weather is fine. Other steps that can help are

- closing the bathroom door to stop steam spreading to
  other rooms
- making sure tumble-dryers are vented to the outside
- putting lids on pans when cooking.

Major indoor air pollutants

Pollutant	Sources	Health Effects
Ammonia	Blueprint machines, cleaning solutions	Respiratory system, eye and skin irritation
Abestos	Duct and pipe insulation, spackling compounds, insulation products, fire retardants, ceiling and floor tiles	Pulmonary (lung) fibrosis, cancer
Benzene	Synthesic fibres, plastics, cleaning solutions, tobacco smoke	Central nervous system damage, skin, respiratory system irritant. Possibly genetic damage
Carbon dioxide	Humans' exhaled air, combustion	Headache, nausea, dizziness
Carbon monoxide	Automotive exhaust, tobacco smoke, combustion	Headache, weakness, dizziness, nausea, long-term exposure related to heart disease
Ethanol	Duplicating fluids	Dermatitis, liver damage, intoxication
Fibreglass	Insulation material	Skin irritations, possible lung damage
Formaldehyde	Urea-formaldehyde foam insulation and urea-formaldehyde resin used to bind laminated wood products such as particle board and plywood; tobacco smoke	Respiratory system, eye and skin irritation, nausea, headache, fatigue, cancer (in exposed laboratory animals)
Methyl alcohol	Spirit duplicating machines	Respiratory system and skin irritation
Micro-organisms (such as viruses, bacteria and fungi)	Humidifying and air-conditioning systems, evaporative condensers, cooling towers, mildewed papers, old books, damp newsprint	Respiratory infection, allergic responses

Fig.4 Pollutants in the air

Motor vehicle exhaust (carbon monoxide, nitrogen oxides, lead particulates, sulphur oxides)	Parking garages, outside traffic	Respiratory system and eye irritation, headache (see carbon monoxide), genetic damage
Nitogen oxides	Gas stoves, combustion, motor vehicle exhaust, tobacco smoke	Respiratory system and eye irritation
Ozones	Photocopying and other electrical machines	Respiratory system and eye irritation, headache, genetic damage
Paint fumes (organics, lead, mercury)	Freshly painted surfaces	Respiratory system and eye irritation; neurological, kidney, and bone marrow damage at high levels of exposure
Pesticides	Spraying of plants, premises	Depending on chemical components: liver damage, cancer, neurological damage, skin, respiratory system and eye irritation
Radon and decay products	Buildings construction materials such as concrete and stone; basements	Ionizing radiation-related diseases such as genetic damage, cancer, foetal and sperm damage
Sterilant gases (such as ethylene oxide)	Systems to sterilize humidifying and air-conditioning systems	Depending on chemical components: respiratory system and eye irritation, genetic damage, cancer
Tobacco smoke (passive exposure to particulates, carbon monoxide, formaldehyde, coal tars, and nicotine)	Cigarettes, pipes, cigars	Respiratory system and eye irritation; may lead to diseases associated with smokers; low-birthweight babies; contributes to poor sperm count
Toluene	Rubber cements, cleaning fluids	Narcotic, skin irritant

Source: General, Municipal, Boilermakers and Allied Trades Union.

ventilation, but it may also be necessary to wear protective breathing equipment.

At home

Perhaps the biggest cause of asthma, and the most common, is the now almost legendary *house dust mite*. This minute but gruesome-looking creature – so small it is (thankfully) invisible to the human eye – is an eight-legged 'carnivore' related to the spider family. On average only a third of a millimetre long it lives on scales of dead human skin and thrives in the static environment of the modern centrally-heated double-glazed home.

Mites occur literally in their millions in most of our houses, particularly in bedding where they live on the flakes of skin we shed while we sleep. Most of us, unknowingly, spend about eight hours every night in close contact with them. It is the mite's droppings – approximately the size of pollen grains – to which some people are allergic. The droppings become easily airborne from the normal tossing and turning in bed as well as when beds are made and are then just as easily inhaled. One estimate has put the number of dust mites in a double mattress and pillows at about two million, with the females laying about 50 eggs a day!

Getting rid of the mite

You can take the following steps to help reduce the level of house dust mites but it is unlikely you will get rid of them completely:

- Buy a new mattress and cover it with a special barrier. Manufacturers have not been slow to develop fabrics that claim to be able to keep out mites. You should find them in most leading stores.
- Cover or replace all carpets with plastic flooring and small, washable rugs, if needed. Nylon carpets are

better than woollen ones for reducing the level of airborne 'allergens' (substances that can trigger an allergic reaction, such as asthma).

- Wash or vacuum clean your carpets regularly. Chemicals known as *acaricides* can kill house dust mites but the droppings remain in carpets which must be vacuumed. Liquid nitrogen can also kill mites in beds and soft furnishings but droppings, too, must be removed by vacuuming. Cleaners for dry vacuuming carpets and soft furnishings have been developed that are highly effective at removing allergen particles. Again, in most developed countries they are readily available at leading stores. In the UK the Consumers' Association has recommended the following as being the best:
- Medivac Microfilter M02
- AEG Compact Electronic 406
- Deluxe 607.

In Britain, you can get further information about environmental control from the British Allergy Foundation (see Appendix A).

Family support
Illnesses can spark off conflict within the family – for example, between parents when, say, the mother devotes a lot of time to the sick child and neglects her husband, or among brothers and sisters who may also resent the constant attention the sick child is getting. But researchers are now starting to look into whether the opposite is also true: that members of a sufferer's family may be able to help prevent an attack in the first place.

Dr David Mrazek, head of psychiatry at the Children's National Medical Center in Washington DC, for example, is running a study to see if family members of asthmatics can effectively intervene to prevent an attack. His study is looking at four different approaches covering all the main risk factors connected to the early onset of asthma. So:

- families in one group are visited regularly by a lay person who helps them to cope with stress factors
- another group is given dietary advice for feeding their new baby

---

Helping children

Parents of asthmatic children (or even potentially asthmatic children) can help them avoid attacks by the following actions:

- Mothers should try to breast-feed for the first 12 months, particularly if there is a history of allergies in the family. There is evidence that breast-fed babies are more resistant to allergies than others (probably because mothers' milk contains the chemicals that help the development of a healthy immune system) and breast-feeding may at least delay and reduce symptoms.
- Damp-dust children's bedroom regularly and wash bedclothes every week on a fast coloureds/white nylon wash at 60°C. Mites can be eliminated from pillows by putting them in the deep-freeze for six hours. Air bedclothes daily.
- Once a fortnight put soft toys in a plastic bag and leave them overnight in the deep-freeze. Then comb all the furry parts with a fine comb.
- Supply children who suffer severe asthma attacks with a peak-flow meter to warn them when they are overdoing any particular physical activity (see box 'Checking your asthma' on page 45).
- If your children sleep in bunk beds let the one with asthma have the top bunk.
- Encourage children to keep away from roads where there is a lot of traffic and pollution levels are likely to be high. (Parents could help further by campaigning for the strict monitoring of pollution levels and the implementation of measures to reduce pollution if not eliminate it altogether.)

- a third group is given both help in coping with stress factors and dietary advice, and
- the fourth and final group is given only an educational session about risk factors for the development of asthma.

The research could decide a great deal about many of the areas currently uncertain about the prevention of asthma and the results are eagerly awaited by many workers in the field. But in the meantime there is still plenty that can be done.

Self-help treatment by methods not involving drugs is mainly a matter of sensible eating and exercise. But there are at least some specific steps you can take:

Exercise and movement
Though some forms of exercise can sometimes aggravate and even precipitate asthma, exercise is generally something to encourage in the right conditions and circumstances. Exercise encourages the heart and lungs to work and so helps boost the body's immune system, the body's own natural built-in system for defeating disease of all sorts.

The benefits of exercise to someone with asthma are many:

- It improves the efficiency and capacity of the heart and lungs.
- It improves circulation, both from the heart end and the muscle end.
- It improves mobility and agility.
- It improves the body's ability to cope with stress.
- It lowers blood pressure.
- It provides more energy to keep you going for longer periods.
- It prevents tiredness and improves concentration.
- It allows the physical expression of buried feelings.
- It removes stale air from the lungs.

Lack of exercise, the poor posture and the stooped shoulders of the asthmatic in which the lungs are pulled in, and a lifestyle that involves spending hours inside (watching TV, for example, or playing with computer games) will almost inevitably lead to shallow breathing. The British yoga teacher Howard Kent says: 'Shallow breathing often results in only the air in the top of the lungs being changed. The lower lobes tend to retain only stale air. This not only limits breathing but reduces the capacity of the lungs to work.' (See also chapter 7.)

Most doctors will say the answer isn't to give up exercise but to take the right medication just before the exercise begins. The natural therapist, on the other hand, is more likely to recommend gentle exercise, such as yoga, including diaphragmatic breathing exercises, or *Ta'i Chi Chu'an*, which accomplishes control of mind and body through slow and rhythmical movements. Posture is also important. This can be practised without undue effort. Even walking in a way that exercises the muscles without straining them is good exercise.

Swimming

Swimming, particularly in heated swimming pools where the warm air does not irritate, is probably the best form of exercise for asthmatics. The exercise of swimming with its breathing control is very helpful. If you swim rhythmically without exertion you will establish a rhythmical way of deep breathing which is one of the best ways of strengthening and relaxing the lungs. Regular swimming can do as much for you as any exercise.

Although an indoor swimming pool is best for asthmatics, particularly in cold weather countries like Britain, swimming in the sea can provide bracing exercise and sea-breezes can also bring relief. But water that is too cold may trigger an attack, as can water (and beaches) that are polluted. Check the beach is safe before you use it! In the UK, where the standard of beaches has come in for considerable criticism from the European Commission, the *Good Beach Guide* (Ebury Press) gives a useful idea of the state of most coastal resorts.

Checking your asthma

One of the most useful pieces of equipment for sufferers is the peak-flow meter. The meter measures lung capacity and is used in diagnosing asthma. It works by measuring the maximum speed at which air can flow *out* of the lungs, known as the *peak expiratory flow rate* (PEFR). It is useful in assessing the severity of constriction (or *bronchospasm*) because narrowed airways slow the rate at which air is expelled. Not everybody needs one but it can be a powerful psychological boost to some people just to have one handy, even preventing an attack that way. They are light and easy to carry and can be used to monitor the state of your airways at different times of the day and from day to day. This will help give an indication of how 'twitchy' your airways are. Children can be easily taught to use them to monitor lung capacity before and during prolonged physical activity. It will warn a child if he or she is heading for a breathing crisis. The meter can be bought (or ordered) from most leading pharmacists.

Eating and drinking

A good diet for asthma sufferers as well as those who suffer from allergies generally is a diet that is good for anyone: that is, one that is not too high in either protein or fat or too low in fibre. Unfortunately many people in the west favour diets that are exactly those things.

Healthy eating and drinking is really only a matter of remembering three simple 'laws':

- eat a wide variety of foods
- eat a little of each
- eat not too much of any.

Some asthma sufferers, however, may not be able to eat certain foods – for example, dairy products. But a healthy diet does not have to include dairy products or even meat and it need not be boring. There are any number of cookbooks available with healthy diets, including vegetarian or diabetic cookbooks, full of the most mouth-watering ideas for meals.

Parents of an asthmatic child should aim to plan meals that are not only good for the child but also acceptable to everyone in the family and to visitors. The sort of food that is good for you – which could include meat, fish, fruit and vegetables – is the sort that has been

---

Tips for reducing pesticides

Some pesticides used in food production are asthma triggers so to avoid them you should:

● wash fruit and vegetables thoroughly before cooking or using in salads.

● remove the outer layers of leafy vegetables such as cabbages or lettuces. (This should get rid of the worst-affected parts. When vegetables are sprayed with chemicals any residue will tend to concentrate on the outer surface. It is estimated that about 90 per cent of lettuces are treated in this way.)

● scrub fruit and vegetables to get rid of pesticide residues, and skin fruit if you can't wash it. (Always wash fruit you buy from a stall or shop, especially if it is on a main road with petrol fumes and other pollutants in the air. Don't throw away the skin if you can possibly help it because it contains valuable nutrients.)

● grow your own food without chemical treatments (but remember that there may be chemical residues in your soil you can't control so it is still best to wash all fruit and vegetables thoroughly before use. This applies just as much to 'organic' food as any other because there is no agreed definition about what organic means and fewer controls over producers making such claims.)

enjoyed by families for centuries. Foods that are not so good are those introduced in only the last 20 to 30 years or so: fatty hamburgers and French fries, for example.

Many sorts of food and drink, including food additives (colourings and preservatives) as well as drugs, are triggers for asthma and adult asthmatics would do well to get into the habit of examining the labels of packaged foods bought in a supermarket. Among the worst additive offenders are *tartrazine* (E102) and *sunset yellow* (E110) used as yellow colouring in pastries, cakes, cordials and squashes. Though not chemically related to aspirin they seem to act in the same way. (About five per cent of asthmatics are affected by aspirin so it is very important to know if you are an 'aspirin asthmatic'.)

Another ingredient commonly used in drinks and food is *sulphur dioxide*. It is used as a preservative in meats and in some wines and beers as well as soft drinks. Alcoholic drinks very often appear in lists of asthma triggers for this reason. Experts point out that many times more people are allergic to foods than food additives, however.

'Reactions to milk, eggs, fish and peanuts are infinitely more common' [than to food additives], says Professor John Warner, a British specialist in child health. It is for this reason he advises asthma sufferers to find out exactly what foods they are allergic to if they can and always to carry around medicines that will help them if they accidently eat one of those foods.

It is not always obvious from the packaging that the food contains the allergic substance. This can sometimes even apply to so-called healthfood snacks. The result can be fatal. In a recent case in the UK a girl died after eating a meringue pie made, unknown to her, with peanuts to which she was fatally allergic.

Beware special diets Most diets are beneficial if

followed sensibly and correctly (even if some conventionally-trained dieticians object) but many can also result in deficiencies in some important vitamins and minerals such as zinc and the 'anti-allergy' vitamins B6 and B12. They can, however, be replaced simply by taking food supplements. A good multi-vitamin tablet once a day would do it (see also chapter 7). There is more on special diets for asthmatics in chapter 7.

Food supplements
Certain foods supplements are recommended for their anti-allergic properties. They include cod liver oil, oil of evening primrose and the B-complex vitamins. Both cod liver oil and evening primrose oil are what are known as *essential fatty acids* (EFAs).

American immunologist Leo Galland believes that asthma may actually be the result of a slight malfunction of the immune system as a result of an imbalance of fatty acids. He has cited several studies showing that children with asthma have difficulty converting EFAs into *prostaglandins* which regulate the working of the immune system. Prostaglandins are controlled by enzymes.

In a special 1993 report in the campaigning UK newsletter *What Doctors Don't Tell You* Galland says: 'If an effective allergy desensitization technique is used, and as much environmental control as possible is exercised, drug-free treatment is virtually always possible in children.' He recommends parents should add the following supplements to their children's diet:

- High doses of essential fatty acids: one tablespoon of linseed (flaxseed) oil and one tablespoon of cod-liver oil.
- Magnesium (3mg per pound of body weight per day).
- Calcium (600mg per day if dairy products are eliminated).

- High doses of vitamin C (2gms a day), B6 (at least 200mg a day), and B12: (1mg twice a day for six weeks).

Summary

For those with allergic asthma an important step in planning your own personal self-help programme is, of course, to establish exactly what foods and substances you are allergic to and to what degree. To do this quickly and accurately it is usually best to consult an experienced clinical ecologist or allergist. The names of organizations that could help with recommendations are in Appendix A.

You can also help yourself by thinking about what you can do to help others. In every illness fellow-sufferers can tell you a lot that doctors can't. So talk to them. Join a group, not just seeking help but as someone who has something positive to offer. Your own experience is your greatest strength. Share it with others.

CHAPTER 5

Conventional treatments and procedures

What your doctor is likely to tell you

Conventional treatment for asthma concentrates on the use of specific drugs known as *corticosteroids* and *beta-antagonists*. Most doctors will recommend one of two main types of drug medication (see box opposite):

● Preventers
● Relievers.

Doctors' attitude and the 'placebo effect'
Most doctors tell their patients it is necessary to take drugs as a matter of routine because without proper control lungs may become permanently damaged. They maintain that with a positive mental attitude and good medical help asthma can be beaten. A key question in asthma is how much is the positive attitude and how much is the medication responsible for successful treatment?

Michael Balint, author of the classic *The Doctor, the Patient and his Illness*, said that of all the therapeutic agents used in medicine, the one in most common use was one about which we had least information. It was not mentioned in the textbooks of medicine, no data existed about the correct dosage, method of use and frequency of administration, or of the allergic or toxic side-effects. He was referring, of course, to the doctor or therapist himself or herself!

Preventers

Drugs to prevent asthma work by building up a protection in the linings of the airways that makes them less likely to narrow when triggered. But they only work if taken regularly and can take a little time (from a few days to a few weeks) to be fully effective.

They come mainly in two types: inhaled steroids and oral steroids (though they can also be injected). Inhaled steroids are claimed to produce less side-effects than the sometimes quite severe ones noted with oral steroids. This is because only very small doses are used and the inhaler delivers the drug particles straight to the lung where they are needed. But even so, among the side-effects reported are hoarseness, fungal infections in the throat, tension and palpitations. Examples of preventive drugs are:

Trade name	Chemical name
Intal	Sodium cromoglycate
Pulmicort	Budesonide
Tilade	Nedocromil sodium
Various	Beclomethasone dipropionate

Relievers

These drugs relieve asthma symptoms very quickly. They are taken as soon as symptoms appear and act mainly on the muscles surrounding the airways, relaxing them and opening them up. Reliever drugs are also most often used with an inhaler – known as a 'blue inhaler' – but they can be taken as tablets or, particularly by very young children, as a syrup. The efect of taking relievers by inhaler lasts for about four hours. Tablets which release the drug slowly over a period have a longer lasting effect. They are recommended for symptoms occuring at night.

Medicines for the relief of asthma also come in two groups: quick-acting drugs and slower-acting drugs that must be taken regularly, like preventers, to be effective. The most commonly reported side-effect is hand tremor.

Examples are:	
Trade name	*Chemical name*
Quick-acting	
Bricanyl	Terbutaline
Ventolin	Salbutamol
Slow-acting	
Atrovent	Ipratropium bromide
Phyllocontin Continus	Aminophylline
Theo-dur	Theophylline

It is a fact, in other words, that people are helped to get well because they believe in a treatment or a practitioner. But sometimes no amount of belief, or treatment, helps. Asthma is a life-threatening condition and in emergency situations few doubt that drugs, particularly of the reliever type, are a vital part of the treatment of asthma. The worrying thing about asthma, though, is that in spite of the fact that effective drugs have been available for many years asthma is not decreasing. In fact the opposite is happening: its incidence is rising.

Air pollution is commonly believed to be the main reason for the virtual epidemic being recorded in almost all medically advanced countries. But in the introduction to this book the startling fact was reported that New Zealand, not noted for its air pollution, has more asthma sufferers per head of population than in any other developed country. This has led many researchers to look closer at the drugs themselves to see if they might not be at least partly to blame.

Problems of over-medication

The facts are now starting to emerge. Recently researchers in New Zealand have proved, for example, that frequent use of the bronchodilator *Fenoteril* is extremely dangerous. They now believe that over-use of bronchodilators, the drugs that widen airways, may be responsible for the surprising statistics in the country.

Their work is being looked at by researchers in other countries and in 1993 the British National Asthma Campaign agreed that there is evidence of overuse. In its summer newsletter it stated that the possible repeated use of such bronchodilators as *Ventolin* and *Bricanyl* might be harmful to the heart and circulation. Researchers believe this may be one explanation for the high rate of deaths that occur during severe asthma attacks. Dr John Connell, who took part in the research, now says that *Ventolin* and *Bricanyl* may prove to be 'less useful than orginally thought'. A small study by Canadian researchers reported in the prestigious international medical journal the *Lancet* in October 1993 confirmed these doubts.

Problems with steroids
Most chest physicians push the use of steroids to suppress inflammation. British allergists Drs John Mansfield and David Freed have, however, pointed out three main snags to the use of steroids:

● even the inhaled variety can be dangerous
● they don't always work, especially when the inflammation is not caused by an immune response but by direct toxicity ('poisoning')
● not all mucus is caused by inflammation: it can also be stimulated directly by certain plant toxins called *lectins*.

The 'fear factor'
British family doctor Duncan Keeley has pointed out that asthma varies enormously in its severity and impact - both between people and over time in the same person. Claiming that there is a great deal of 'unnecessary intervention' for people with mild asthma, he comments:

'Doctors need to be able to vary the fuss they make about it'. They might be more successful, he says, if they made light of the diagnosis. He suggests doctors should be 'less threatening and less intrusive and make less fuss about the symptoms'.

Dr Keeley was recognizing that fear is an important component in the disease. Fear aggravates the bronchospasm. This seems to be the nub of the problem. A gentle approach, favoured by complementary therapists, and many doctors too, means paying more attention to the patient as well as to the illness.

As we have stressed in previous chapters, there is a two-way link between asthma and psychological problems. Having a chronic illness such as asthma can be stressful and symptoms associated with the disease can lead to depression or anger. Conversely, depression and anger can aggravate the condition. It has also been found that the disease itself can condition a patient to expect an attack in certain circumstances. For instance, an argument with a partner can trigger an attack – and so a patient may begin to wheeze even before the next argument happens, out of the very fear of conflict itself. The wheeze may even be a psychological response to gain sympathy and avoid conflict.

Summary

The usual way of dealing with an attack of asthma is to reach for a steroid inhaler. For many, the inhaler is a handy way of preventing an asthmatic attack – but it does not tackle the root cause of the problem. It merely relieves the symptoms. This is very useful at times – and at times it is vital – but it is not, of course, a cure. The key to the proper understanding, and treatment, of asthma seems to be in developing an approach which is very much in keeping with the so-called 'holistic' philosophy of the natural therapies. Let's look at them next and see how they can help.

CHAPTER 6

The natural therapies and asthma

Prevention and treatment by the 'gentle alternatives'

In June 1993 the British Medical Association (BMA) published a landmark report in which it conceded for the first time not only that natural therapies (the BMA called them 'non-conventional' therapies) are here to stay but also that some of them should, and probably would, become more widely available to everyone, including the patients of conventional doctors trained in western medical approaches.

In fact, as critics have pointed out, the BMA was only bowing to the inevitable. What it said should happen was already happening: an increasing number of people are seeking help from non-conventional medical practitioners. The trend, the BMA admitted, reflects 'a genuine public need.' But what exactly are these therapies and how do they differ from the conventional medical approach? Why do people go to natural therapists? Most important, which therapies are useful for asthma and how can you find a therapist you can rely on? In this chapter, and in rest of the book, we'll look at the answers to all these questions.

Why go to a natural therapist?

People often turn to a natural therapist as a last resort. They have tried the conventional route and it hasn't worked. For whatever reason – and it may be because their problem was not helped or, sadly, perhaps even made worse – their needs haven't been met. An official report in Israel in 1991 concluded that people there were turning in growing numbers to natural medicine for exactly the same reasons they are turning to it the world over: that is, a concern, even outright disillusionment, over an increasingly specialized and rigid medical profession that is slow to respond not only to the fast-changing nature and incidence of disease in a safe and gentle way – preferring synthetic substances and high technology over 'natural' approaches – but also to the public's growing demand for greater freedom of choice in healthcare and a say in how they are treated.

Whatever the reasons people go to practitioners of natural therapy they seem to get a high level of satisfaction when they do. In Britain, for example, where no therapist is legally required to train to practice non-medical therapy, surveys in recent years have consistently shown satisfaction levels between 60 and 80 per cent. So who are these therapists and what is it about them that appeals so much? What is natural therapy and most important of all, how do you find the right practitioner?

What is natural therapy?

There is a quite a discussion (not to say argument, even among natural therapists themselves) about whether all natural therapies operate under one common idea or principle. The British Medical Association, in its 1993 report, said they did not – that the natural therapies were a mixture of different styles and techniques with nothing in common at all. In fact the natural approaches all understand, accept and operate under the following principles:

- The body has a natural ability to heal itself.
- The human being is not simply a physical machine, like a car, but a subtle and complex blend of body, mind and emotions (or spirit or soul as some prefer to call it) and that all or any of these factors may cause or contribute to problems of health. In other words, that every individual is not a random collection of moving parts but a fully integrated 'whole' (the term 'holistic medicine' has been coined to describe treating the individual as a 'whole being' composed of body, mind and spirit).
- Environmental and social conditions can be just as important as a person's physical and psychological makeup and may have just as big an impact on their health.
- Treating the root cause or causes of a problem is more important than treating the obvious immediate symptoms. Treating only symptoms may simply cover up the real underlying problem and make it worse, so that it reappears later as something more serious.
- Each person is unique and cannot therefore be treated in exactly the same way as every other person.
- Healing is quicker and more effective if the person takes responsibility for his or her own health and has an active involvement in the healing process (but a good therapist will also recognize when someone needs to 'let go' and place themselves in the hands of another).
- Good health is a state of emotional, mental, spiritual and physical 'balance'. (Balance is fundamental to the basic notion of health in natural therapy. Ill-health, say its exponents, is the result of being in a state of

imbalance, or 'dis-ease'. The Chinese express this as the principle of *yin* and *yang*).

● There is a natural healing 'force' in the universe (what the Chinese call *qi* or *chi* – pronounced 'chee' – the Japanese *ki*, Indians *prana* and westerners *vis medicatrix naturae* or 'life force'). Anyone can 'tap into' or make use of this force and it is a natural health practitioner's skill to activate it in the patient or help the patient activate it in themselves.

It is natural therapists' belief in the 'Oriental' ideas expressed particularly in the last two principles – and also often their use of those terms – that have caused so much controversy among so many doctors trained in the western scientific method. It is frequently the single most important reason they reject so much of it. (The reaction is probably understandable given the length of time they have spent in learning a very different system but the principles are there whether they like them or not. Moreover a blanket rejection of all therapies because of a refusal to accept, say, the concept of *qi* – 'life force' – stands the risk of throwing away something that may be beneficial simply because of a dislike of the trappings: the baby with the bathwater syndrome. The important thing is not to be put off just because some doctors get all huffy about it. They may be wrong!).

The essence of all natural therapies, however, is the same and returns very much to the earliest principles of medicine followed, practiced and preached by the ancient healers of Greece and Egypt: that the best approach is the one that is the softest and gentlest, that avoids dangerous and traumatic procedures, that treats the patient as a 'whole' individual, and in which the patient takes an active part in his or her own recovery and health maintenance.

How do natural therapies treat asthma?

Nature's way of dealing with an illness is to try to heal the whole person in body, mind and 'spirit' and equally, as we have seen, the main theme of natural medicine is that all systems influence each other. The natural approach to asthma, as to any other illness, is the gentle one. It is one that sees the illness as part of a general pattern of maladjustment of mind-body processes and not as something that exists as a separate pathological condition or disease that suddenly and mysteriously invades your body and can then be precisely and objectively defined and given a label. A diseased organ exists in the whole person; a sick person exists within a particular social and physical environment.

What the natural therapist has to decide is what is the most appropriate level where intervention may be necessary and can be achieved without side-effects – that is, without damaging any other part of the body/mind – and what methods, or combination of methods, are likely to be most effective.

The natural therapist or practitioner draws together a number of related factors involved in the illness, which may be physical, psychological, genetic, environmental or social. He or she may decide that different skills are needed in the treatment of various aspects of an illness. In the case of asthma, for example, an acupuncturist, an osteopath, a psychotherapist and a clinical ecologist may each have something different and important to offer.

The following natural therapies have been found to benefit asthma in varying ways and to varying degrees (they are described in more detail in chapters 7-9):

- acupuncture
- Alexander Technique
- aromatherapy
- biofeedback

- chiropractic
- counselling/psychotherapy
- healing/Therapeutic Touch
- herbal medicine
- homoeopathy
- hydrotherapy
- hypnotherapy
- massage
- naturopathic medicine
- nutritional therapy/dietary therapy
- osteopathy
- reflexology
- relaxation therapy
- shiatsu
- yoga.

Quite apart from the benefit that may be derived from these specific therapies, there is the common-sense approach (often handed down from generation to generation in families that enjoy good health) in which the patient is responsible for himself or herself. He or she does not have to be told to take exercise, eat wisely, play music, paint, walk, dance, not to smoke or drink heavily and not to overwork. They do these things quite naturally. Coupled with this are the family folk remedies that are also handed down from one generation to the next. A number of modern drugs – a classic example is *digitalis* (from foxglove) used in treating heart conditions – were developed from folk remedies based on a purely word-of-mouth tradition.

As there are multiple factors contributing to the onset of asthma so there must be multiple factors that can lead to a restoration of health. We'll look at how the different therapies listed above can help asthma in the following chapters. Each chapter considers the therapies from the way they mainly work. Therapies such as chiropractic and osteopathy, for example, work principally on the body so are obviously 'physical therapies'. They are dealt with in chapter 7. Techniques such as psychotherapy and hypnotherapy, on the other hand, are all to do with mind and emotions, or the psychology of the person. They are covered in chapter 8. Some therapies operate at all levels – affecting mind and emotions as well as the body – and since many are among those therapies that deal with the 'energy', or 'subtle body' (as it is sometimes also called), of a person there is a separate chapter 9 for them.

The medicine of the future?

As long ago as 1956 a committee of the British Medical Association, set up at the request of the Archbishops' Commission on Divine Healing, published a report which stated: 'Since man is a unity and health a condition of full functioning, we cannot afford, especially in critical illnesses, to disregard any means at our disposal which may lead to the restoration of health, since all the functions of the personality [mind and body] react upon one another.'

It has been said that medicine advances rapidly but changes only slowly. New insights about diseases that have baffled us in the past, such as asthma, are leading only gradually to an improved attitude towards the art of healing. But there is some reason for optimism. One of the discoveries of medical science is that many ancient remedies described in the past as 'fringe medicine' have now been found to have a scientific basis and have become accepted. Acupuncture is a good example.

The examples in the following chapters are quite likely to find a place in the healing of the future before much longer for the same reason.

For how to find and choose a natural therapist see chapter 10.

CHAPTER 7

Treating your body

Physical therapies for asthma

Some natural therapies helpful against asthma treat your body in a directly physical way. That is, they are not concerned with your background psychological condition as much as your immediate physical symptoms. In this sense natural therapies are closest to conventional medicine in that they are sometimes treating symptoms rather than underlying causes, but at least they aim to do so in the gentlest way possible, without drugs and without side-effects. Moreover the effect of such therapies is often, by working from the outside in as it were, to remove the underlying causes anyway.

Therapies that have been shown to be beneficial in cases of asthma come under the following general headings:

- manipulation (chiropractic and osteopathy)
- massage (aromatherapy)
- medication (Western and Chinese herbal medicine)
- movement (yoga)
- naturopathic medicine (hydrotherapy)
- nutritional/dietary therapy.

Manipulation

Posture is important in maintaining health. According to

practitioners who specialize in the manipulation of the muscles and bones of the body (the 'musculo-skeletal system') such as osteopaths and chiropractors, for example, a structural or mechanical defect is often present in cases of asthma. People with lung complaints tend to be round-shouldered with a distended chest. Manipulators claim to have found small displacements in the rib-cage and the area of the spine that supports the ribs. The 'asthmatic pattern' of tense, round chest, neck, shoulders and diaphragm are all areas that can be dealt with effectively by manipulation.

Alexander Technique

The Alexander Technique (AT) is not really a therapy nor does it require the services of a therapist to administer it, but it is about the correct use of muscles and bones – in particular the muscles and bones of the head and shoulders. The technique, devised in the 1920s by an Australian actor called F. Matthias Alexander who had breathing and speaking problems, is a way of learning how to 'educate' your head to sit in correct alignment with your spine. Its aim is to get rid of bad habits and to restore the body to its natural way of moving. Alexander's famous saying was: 'When you stop doing the wrong thing, the right thing does itself.' It is really a self-help method you can practise for yourself once you have learned it from a trained teacher.

AT is a classic 'outside-in' exercise, with improvements to posture leading to improvements in mood, stability and health and well-being generally. As well as curing many of the aches and pains that come from bad posture and movement the technique can, like many other forms of exercise, help to lower blood pressure, solve digestive trouble and improve breathing. It has helped asthmatics.

Alexander Technique relaxation exercise

The object of this simple exercise is to relax the body and allow it to be free of tension. Lie on a hard surface with the legs apart (about shoulder width), knees bent, and the head resting on two or three paperback books, not a pillow. The bony hump at the back of the head (known as the *occiput*), not the neck, should be resting on the books as in the illustration below. The arms should be placed with the elbows on the floor and the palms of the hands across the midriff. Stay like this for about 20 minutes. As you lie there imagine your shoulders spreading, your spine being pulled down and straightened by gravity, your head growing upwards and outwards. If you keep this up every day, you will find that your spine will straighten and all the bones and muscles in your body will feel right and tensions will go.

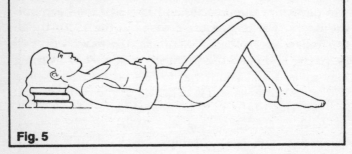

Fig. 5

Chiropractic

The word 'chiropractic' is derived from a Greek word meaning 'manual practice.' Osteopathy and chiropractic work in almost the same way, the main difference being historical. Both systems were developed by American practitioners at the end of the last century but the founder of osteopathy, Andrew Taylor Still, claimed that blood supply was the essential factor in healthy tissue whereas David Daniel Palmer, the founder of chiropractic, emphasized nerves. Today both practices treat the same complaints using mainly manipulation techniques to correct tensions and imbalances in the musculo-skeletal system. Both claim to be able to treat asthma successfully.

In America, both techniques are well established with around 30,000 chiropractors and 20,000 osteopaths. The main difference is that osteopathy in America is practised exclusively by medical doctors. Outside America osteopathy is the more common and it is used mainly by non-medical, although highly qualified, practitioners. But worldwide chiropractic is by far the bigger profession, larger in fact than all other natural therapies together.

CHIROPRACTIC: James Robinson's story

James Robinson, 4, suffered from both asthma and eczema and was allergic to certain foods and animals. His asthma was never serious enough to put him into hospital but he needed to take steroids (*Becotide*) and a bronchodilator (*Salbutamol*) fairly regularly during the winter months each year.

His mother Anne, who was being treated for a whiplash injury asked her chiropractor if she could do anything for James. The chiropractor had never treated asthmatics before but said she believed chiropractic could be of some help and so treatment began.

The chiropractor diagnosed a problem in his lower neck and upper thoracic spine and treated James using a combination of gentle manipulation and an activator (a mechanical means of manipulation).

James developed a chest infection soon after starting treatment, for which he was given antibiotics. To his mother's surprise this did not trigger his asthma as it would have done before the treatment. The slightest cold used to precipitate an attack.

After five months of treatment James was free of asthma and his twice-daily peak flow readings had been reduced to intermittent.

Osteopathy

The physical symptoms of asthma may respond well to osteopathic manipulation of the spine, rib-cage and skull. Osteopathy is based on the principle that structure and function are interdependent in the human body in the same way as in an efficient machine. Osteopaths believe that if there is any alteration in the structure of the body it is bound to affect its function. Similarly, if the body is forced to perform a function it was not designed for there will be changes of structure.

OSTEOPATHY: James Tweedle's story

James Tweedie developed asthma at the age of four. His mother, a west London family doctor, believed it was triggered by a combination of allergic and emotional factors. Four years of orthodox treatment, plus a number of sessions with an acupuncturist and hypnotist, hadn't been any help so his mother decided to send him for osteopathic treatment at the British School of Osteopathy's clinic in central London.

He had weekly sessions, in which the osteopath paid special attention to the skull, neck, rib-cage and spine. Within five months his asthma was cured – together with an unexpected bonus: a dramatic increase in his height. The osteopath helped the boy's body to function normally in response to stress. It no longer reacted to emotional stimuli or allergies with an asthma attack.

After that the mother said he was 'a much nicer person to live with.'

Osteopathy sees disease as a distortion of either structure or function. A person who is tense, for example, builds up layers of tight muscles in the back and this can lead to problems in the spine. Children learn to deal with feelings in different ways, and in adapting to adult standards of behaviour they sometimes hold onto their emotions by becoming more tense in the body. Spinal manipulation of children affected in this way, which can include asthma sufferers, may be one way of tackling the problem. But osteopaths don't just 'crack' joints, they massage too.

Tensions in muscles of the back can be relieved by soft-tissue massage. One such method, for example, is the 'neuro-muscular technique' (NMT). It consists of deep, controlled movement by the balls of the therapist's thumbs or surfaces of the fingers over particular parts of the body connected to the ligaments and muscles of the spine. Once the chest and diaphragm are moving more freely, says the osteopath, symptoms and psychological tension will improve.

Massage

We communicate in many different ways with our bodies – our pleasures as well as our pains and anxieties – as the psychologists Wilhelm Reich and his American pupil Alexander Lowen, founder of 'bioenergetics', have shown. Reich taught about 'body-armouring', which he described as the holding back of 'bioenergy' in the body in various ways, especially in the muscles.

Massage is one of the most direct and obvious ways of releasing body tensions that build up in stressful situations such as an asthma attack. Releasing body tensions can also release mental and emotional tensions (some therapists will say that this is the real purpose of massage) and it is this widely-known and supported fact that has led to massage being one of the most popular and effective of physical therapies.

The variations available are enormous, from the extreme vigour of the famous 'Swedish massage' to techniques like 'Therapeutic Touch' that are so gentle you can hardly feel yourself being touched. (In fact some people even think the gentle touch techniques have more to do with 'hands-on healing' than massage there is so little 'massage' involved.)

Almost all massage techniques are suitable for most asthmatics, provided they are given by a competent person, and the choice is more to do with personal preference and what works best for you in any given situation. One of the most popular these days is aromatherapy.

Aromatherapy
Strictly speaking aromatherapy is not massage at all because the name means simply 'therapy with aromas' or 'smell therapy'. Smell is one of the most powerful of our senses as anyone knows who has had memories of the past recalled vividly for them by a smell. But there is a respectable body of evidence now that specific smells can also help heal. A traditional Indian form of medicine known as *Ayurveda* has used aromas for centuries in the belief they can cure pain and alleviate coughs and colds.

The smells in aromatherapy are based on the distilled oil essences of various plants and herbs, hence the name 'essential oils'. A skilled aromatherapist will use a specific oil or combination of oils to treat a variety of conditions, including asthma. The oils can be inhaled, vaporized, used in hot compresses and even gargled – but it is their use in massage for which they are most popular and best known.

In asthma the choice of essential oils depends on many factors: whether asthma is an allergic response, for example, or whether emotional factors are involved. Bergamot, camomile, clary, lavender, thyme, neroli and rose oil are all said to be beneficial in asthma, being both anti-spasmodic and anti-depressant. Bergamot and lavender are also supposed to be able to clear up chest infections.

If sleep is a problem aromatherapy can help there too. A few drops of one of the oils in the bath or in a small bowl of hot water on the bedside table before going to

bed can do the trick. Some therapists are cautious about
using aromatherapy during an asthmatic attack itself but
at other times they recommend massaging the whole
chest area, with particular emphasis on strokes which
'open out' the chest and shoulders.

Aromatherapists say it works on the mental and emotional levels as well as the physical. Tension interferes
with the lymph circulation which plays such an important part in the immune system. But anything that
reduces tension is bound to help the asthma sufferer.
Although many doctors are sceptical about whether
essential plant oils can have any significant effect on a
condition such as asthma they usually agree that the
massage itself is important. (Doctors themselves usually
only touch patients for clinical reasons. It's left to nurses
to do the hugging and cuddling, particularly of children,
which can sometimes be of more benefit than the medicine!)

Medication

Natural medication, which means the use of herbs to
heal, is the closest natural medicine comes to conventional medicine, and for obvious reasons. Herbs – a term
which applies not just to herbs but to all plants, including ferns, seaweeds, trees and lichens – were the only
remedies prescribed by doctors and folk healers until
quite recent times. It is only since the development of the
chemical industry a century ago that synthetic drugs
have taken over. But even today many modern medicines – about a quarter of all those in use – are derived
from plants used in folk medicine in a tradition handed
down for centuries from generation to generation. This
sort of knowledge is still passed on among the Indian
tribes of rain-forests such as the Amazon – which is one
reason the drugs industry is now starting to learn as

much about the thousands of still undiscovered herbs as they can before they, and the Indians, are destroyed.

The reason herbalists prefer herbs to synthetically extracted drugs, however, is because herbalists believe nature has built-in the right blend of checks and balances in a naturally grown plant that are not there in a single chemical isolated from the rest of the plant. So a herb with a particular active ingredient useful for a specific condition is likely also to have some other ingredients that spontaneously tone down or balance-out any harmful side-effects, making it safer and gentler than a pharmaceutical drug.

Western herbal medicine

Though the use of medicinal herbs faded with the rise of other forms of medicine it never died, particularly in Europe, and today the tradition is becoming popular again, with practitioners in many countries training extensively in the full and proper use of herbal remedies. Such a training is really essential because herbs can be powerful and many are extremely dangerous. An example is foxglove, from which the heart drug *digitalis* is extracted but which is actually poisonous. That is why it is always advisable to consult a fully qualified herbal practitioner for any serious condition such as asthma. Also herbalism has moved on.

A famous European herbalist, the 17th-century British practitioner Nicholas Culpepper, recommended honeysuckle and black horehound with honey for coughs and sore throats as well as breathlessness but no modern herbalist is likely to suggest these herbs for asthma. Simon Mills, one of Britain's leading modern herbalists, mentions only that herbs like grindelia (*grindelia spp*), skunk cabbage (*symptlocarpus foetidus*) and lobelia relieve tension and therefore might be helpful for asthma.

Chinese herbal medicine

The extensive use of herbs is a major part of Traditional Chinese Medicine (TCM) that has been practised for some 2,500 years. It includes acupuncture (see chapter 9). TCM is now being recognized in the West as offering successful treatments for various problems including allergic conditions such as asthma. Doctors at the famous Great Ormond Street Hospital for Sick Children in London, for example, were impressed recently when they saw cases of severe eczema they had been unable to help with modern drugs responding successfully to a special formula of ten Chinese herbs. There is no such known formula for the treatment of asthma yet but Western medicine is now taking a hard and close look at the 2,000 and more herbs used in TCM and some such discovery could follow.

According to Chinese medicine three organs are involved in asthma: the lung, the spleen and the kidney. The main cause is described as 'phlegm'. However a Chinese doctor will not identify the cause and nature of the case until he or she has thoroughly examined the patient and taken an individual history. Some cases respond to kidney tonics but if the trouble is in the spleen or lungs different treatments will be given. Some cases respond either to herbs or acupuncture but not both. On the other hand, there have been cases in which acupuncture triggers an attack in susceptible patients – so it is important, again, it should be administered only by fully-qualified practitioners.

TCM also takes account of a patient's full circumstances, including environmental, family and social factors as well as eating habits (another reminder that the principles of 'holism' are far from new!) and it is common for a practitioner to recommend dietary changes as part of treatment.

Movement

As already mentioned in chapter 4, asthma sufferers can benefit from the right exercise but there are various specific movement and breathing exercises particularly suited to the asthmatic because they teach them to become aware of their body and to listen to 'information signals' about their responses that flow in and out of the body most of the time. The most effective all come from yoga.

Yoga

Yoga is the ancient Indian art of using your body to influence your mind, and therefore your health, through a variety of exercises involving both movement and breathing. Many physical exercises can leave you feeling tired, aching all over and discouraged. But this is not true of yoga.

Yoga is concerned with joining or relating the different parts of the body for the efficient functioning of the *whole* body. But more than anything else it is about balance. In every exercise or posture (*asana*) it is the quality of movement that counts more than the effort that is put into achieving a certain posture.

Many people find the exercises exhilarating and at the same time relaxing. A student who tried many other forms of exercise said that yoga increased her confidence in her own body that many other exercises failed to achieve: 'Far from being the stiff ungainly object that was forever letting me down, I found that my body was strong, dynamic, capable of far more than I ever imagined. It was just a matter of working with it rather than pitting myself against it.'

Yoga and asthma

Yoga has been used to treat patients with asthma for over 50 years in centres in India. The benefits of yoga were demonstrated in a long-term study of 53 patients carried out by doctors at the Vivekananda Kendra Yoga Therapy and Research Centre in Bangalore.

The patients spent two weeks performing under guidance an integrated set of three different sorts of yoga exercise as well as a devotional session. The exercises were:

- physical postures (*suryanamaskar* and *yogasana*)
- slow breathing techniques (*pranayama*), and
- meditation (*dhyana*).

After doing the exercises for 65 minutes every day they were compared with another matching group of 53 asthma patients who had continued to take their usual drugs. It was found that there was a more significant improvement in the group who practised yoga than in the control group.

Yoga breathing

Yoga breathing exercises can be of great benefit to asthmatics. Known as 'complete breathing', yoga breathing consists of three parts: 'abdominal'. 'middle' (rib-cage), and 'upper chest' breathing.

- *Abdominal breathing* This is done standing, sitting or lying. It is best at first to practise lying down with knees bent, because then you can really feel what is happening. Your attention is directed to the region of the navel. You place the palms of the hands over this region while exhaling and emptying your lungs completely. The abdominal wall is drawn in tightly, forcing air out of the lungs through the nose. Then you breathe in slowly through the nose relaxing the diaphragm. The abdominal wall curves outwards and the lower part of the lung fills with air.

- *Middle (rib-cage) breathing* This time your attention is directed to the ribs. Rest the palms of the hands on the rib-cage. After exhaling and emptying the lungs completely inhale slowly through the nose. The ribs expand. When exhaling, the ribs contract and squeeze the air out through the nose. In middle breathing the middle part of the lung is filled with air. The abdomen and shoulders do not move.
- *Upper chest breathing* Your attention is directed to the top of the chest where you place the palms of your hands with fingertips touching. Exhale, emptying your lungs completely. Then breathe in slowly.
- *Complete breathing* Your attention is directed to the whole of your trunk as you follow the wave-like movements of your breathing. Begin with palms placed on the stomach and exhale to empty the lungs. Slowly breathe in through the nose, counting up to eight, sliding the hands upwards as the diaphragm moves down and the rib-cage expands as the lungs fill with air. Exhale, relaxing the diaphragm and sliding the hands down to the stomach. Repeat the exercise with your arms resting at your side. The whole exercise should be experienced in a single movement. The exercise induces a feeling of peace and well-being.

Diaphragmatic release

This exercise is designed to achieve a deep, uninhibited breath and the greatest possible movement of the diaphragm. It is performed sitting on your heels on the floor. You begin by bending forward, as deeply as possible, with the forearms lying flat on the ground, the head quite loose, dangling towards the floor (*see figure 6*).

Breathe out deeply and then as you breathe in, swing up with your arms reaching to the ceiling. Finally sweep downwards breathing out strongly as you collapse with your forearms once more resting on the ground. This

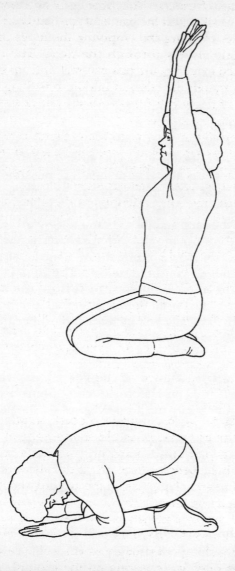

Fig. 6 Breathing exercises

should be repeated, say, a dozen times. The exercises should be done freely, without any straining. You should feel like a floppy doll.

Mountain stretches

This deep-breathing exercise can be performed sitting on the floor. It would be suitable for asthmatics, helping not only with the breathing but also with the stretching of the muscles of the trunk.

Sitting erect, the arms loose by the side, you first of all breathe out. Next breathe in as you stretch the arms out to the sides and up above your head, if possible just behind the line of the shoulder blades to enhance the stretch and lift the muscles of the trunk. The arms should touch the ears, and the maximum upward stretch can be helped by linking the thumbs. After a few seconds the arms are slowly brought down again, stretching all the time as you breathe out. The idea is that breathing and movement should follow the same rhythm. Half a dozen mountain stretches performed slowly and rhythmically will increase lung capacity and strengthen chest and arms.

'Huffing'

Huffing, otherwise known as the Forced Expiration Technique (FET), is an effective technique to help to clear the chest of sticky mucus (see figure 7). The patient takes a normal breath in and then blows hard with some force. The patient is advised to try huffing against a mirror or window pane. If it mists up enough to write on the patient will know he is doing it right.

There are three huffing exercises specially recommended for children:

● Flapping the arms (wings) against the sides as they huff. Small children can pretend to be geese, flapping angrily and hissing.

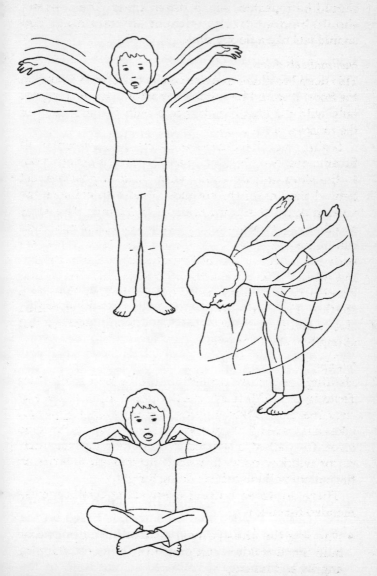

Fig. 7 'Huffing'

- Bending over and swinging the arms from side to side, turning the body in one movement. Swinging movements prevent the rib-cage from stiffening.
- Sitting cross-legged on the floor, touch your shoulders with your fingers. Circle your elbows round and round like back-stroke swimming.

In another breathing out exercise, used by the American pioneers Daniel Brown and Erika Fromm, you begin by breathing normally. Then you put slight but steady emphasis on the expiration as if slightly but gently pushing each breath. At the same time picture yourself pushing out the walls of the room (this is called 'visualization'). Brown and Fromm reported that one patient described this exercise as a way of increasing his 'breathing room.'

Bellows breathing
In 'bellows breathing' you place your hands on your waist above your hips, with the fingers extending slightly over the sides of the stomach and the thumbs slightly over the sides of the back. You are told to focus your attention carefully on how your hands move when you breathe and, specifically, to detect the degree of outward movement (like the bellows expanding sideways). In proper diaphragmatic breathing the main thrust of the hands is forward. You can thus use the hands as a feedback device to train yourself in diaphragmatic breathing.

Naturopathic medicine

Naturopathic medicine, originally known as 'Nature Cure' (and still called that by some), is based on the body's built-in ability to repair itself. In a normally healthy person cuts and wounds heal, fractured bones mend, and germs are exterminated automatically by the body's own defence mechanisms. So naturopathic treatment aims first of all at purifying the system of poisons or 'toxins' it believes get in the way of or undermine this natural process, and then at building up the general health level of the sufferer.

Naturopaths believe asthma is a 'whole person' illness, not just a disorder of the respiratory system. In common with other conditions such as migraine and eczema, whatever the combination of causes, most naturopaths believe a disturbance in the function of the digestive system is fundamental.

The late British naturopath Harry Benjamin, for example, author of *Everybody's Guide to Nature Cure,* believed that this was the main cause of the illness: 'The stomach and bronchi and bronchial tubes are connected by the vagus nerve, and by reflex action digestive disturbance can so affect the bronchi and bronchial tubes that the passage of air through them is restricted, and an asthmatic attack precipitated.

'Obviously a catarrhal condition of the bronchial tubes will tend to make the appearance of asthma more likely than otherwise, and a highly nervous and run-down condition of the system will also lead to its development.'

According to Benjamin 'a thorough internal cleansing of the system and a building-up of the tone of the whole organism' can cure 'the asthma bogey. . . completely in many cases, providing other serious complications do not happen to be present.' Benjamin's treatment involved a short fast, a daily rub with a dry sponge, breathing exercises every night, warm-water enemas, a diet of fruit and fresh vegetables, hot Epsom-salts baths twice a week, and plenty of outdoor exercise.

Modern naturopaths, particularly outside the UK, have adopted a whole range of other therapies, including acupuncture, homoeopathy, herbalism, manipulation, massage and nutritional supplements, which

'nature cure' purists frown on. But one they bo
approve of, and one with known benefit in a number
conditions, including asthma, is hydrotherapy.

Hydrotherapy
Hydrotherapy, which means simply 'water therapy',
one of the oldest systems of healing known. Vario
forms of hydrotherapy are found in almost every cultu
on earth, from steam baths and saunas to cold wat
sprays and salt-water bathing. Swimming became popt
lar only after it was first used for reasons of therap
Health hydros, no longer common in Britain, were onc
everywhere based on natural hot water or 'therma
springs, and in Europe they still are.

Asthma has long been recognized as a conditio
helped outstandingly by a number of forms of hydrothe
apy and in Europe asthma sufferers are routinely pre
scribed visits by doctors to the many thermal spring batl
in use. In France, for example, queues of children suffe
ing from asthma are a common sight during the summe
outside the baths at Le Mont-Dore in the Auvergn
(Information about thermal springs in France can b
obtained from: Promothermes, Centre d'Informatio
Thermales, 48 Bvd Malesherbes, Paris 75008, France.)

Methods anyone can try at home, though, includ
something as simple as a relaxing bath, keeping the tem
perature at about 32-34°C for between 40 and 60 min
utes. An 'Epsom bath' – about 1.5lbs (700g) o
commercial Epsom salts put into a normal bath – is also
beneficial, although it is not recommended for people
with heart trouble or for anyone fasting.

'Steaming' is another effective way of clearing mucu
from the airways of the nose, throat and chest. Steam
heat is more effective than other forms of heat. The kettl
should be about three-quarters full of water and a steady
stream of vapour should be maintained.

Nutritional and dietary therapy

Both nutritional and dietary therapy are closely connected to modern naturopathy, particularly outside the UK, and there are a growing number of therapists who specialize in both. Nutritional therapy concentrates mainly on the the prescription of food supplements whereas dietary therapists advise on special diets. The relevance of both to asthma is clearly established.

Research in Scotland at Aberdeen University's medical school, for example, has recently put the blame for the present asthma epidemic firmly on a poor diet, particularly on not eating enough fresh fruit and vegetables. The theory is that this has lowered people's resistance to allergy diseases generally due to a lack of what are known as 'antioxidant' nutrients. Antioxidant nutrients resist the ageing process and boost the body's natural defence system against disease. The main antioxidants are the vitamins A (beta carotene), C and E, and the minerals zinc, selenium and manganese. The researchers argued that the reduction in the consumption of fresh fruit and vegetables in Britain between 1961 and 1985 was matched by a comparable rise in the number of people suffering from asthma.

Although this does not explain the high incidence of asthma in other countries, where people eat a lot more fresh fruit and vegetables than they do in Britain, it illustrates the importance of nutrition in health.

Among special diets with a good reputation in asthma are:

● *Bircher-Benner allergy diet* The Swiss physician Bircher-Benner, who invented *muesli*, recommended diets that cleared the body of toxins and promoted healthy functioning of all the body's organs. His diets were created before we knew a great deal about food allergies but an allergy diet, created by his daughter, Ruth

Bircher-Benner, concentrated exclusively on plant nutrition. She also recommended supplements to make up for deficiencies of vitamins that can only be had from animal food. Her meals consisted of muesli (for breakfast and sometimes for an evening meal), lots of fruit, raw vegetables and nuts, herb tea, apple juice and vegetarian recipes for cooked meals.

- *Raw food diet* A great deal of the nutrients (vitamins and minerals) in food are lost in cooking. Raw food is not only more nutritious but it also contains more fibre. The main loss in cooking is vitamins A and C but you can retrieve much of this if you use the water from cooking for soups or gravies. The loss of magnesium and iron in cooking vegetables can lead to health problems although supplements, again, can replace these fairly easily. The greatest wastage, however, is of mineral salts. This can range from 10 per cent to as much as 60 per cent of the contents. Raw vegetables, such as carrots, beetroot and parsnips can be grated and mixed to make tasty salads.

- *Vegetarian and vegan diets* There is nothing new about either diet. Vegetarianism is as old as civilization and in many parts of the world not eating meat is part of the way of life. In China Taoist writings state that a meatless diet is essential for a 'healthy soul' and in India neither Buddhists nor Hindus are meat-eaters. Today as many people in the West become vegetarians for health reasons as for reasons of principle. A vegetarian diet is one of the healthiest and safest introductions to eating solids for a small child.

Veganism is just a more strict form of vegetarianism. It involves eating only plant food. Like the Bircher-Benner diet, the vegan diet excludes all meat, fish, eggs and dairy products. Vegans generally eat a great deal of raw food such as fruit, nuts and vegetables.

Vegans and vegetarians sometimes lack essential amino acids and zinc as a result but the vegan diet has been found to be well suited to the asthmatic. But if sufferers decide to follow this diet other sources of food allergy must be rigorously eliminated such as treated tap water. Drink only spring (mineral) water and have no coffee, tea, chocolate, sugar or salt (herbal teas are allowed). Most vegetables can be eaten freely but avoid too many potatoes. Fruit is allowed but not apples or citrus fruit (oranges, grapefruit and so on). The benefits this brings is said to be the result of eliminating common food allergens and altering the body's chemistry of fatty acids.

Why animal fats may be bad for asthmatics

The production of *leukotrienes* that contribute to the allergic reactions sometimes found in asthma, including inflammation of the airways, are derived from *arachidonic acid*, a fatty acid found exclusively in animal products. *Leukotrienes are, in fact, a thousand times more potent than histamine.*

Asthma specialists tend to disapprove of a vegan diet, and sometimes even go so far as to claim it could be dangerous. But according to the Vegan Society in Britain health problems in children as a direct result of the diet are rare and, in fact, a study in Sweden on the effects of a vegan 'exclusion diet' on 24 children with asthma found an improvement in almost all the children after a year.

Summary

The physical therapies described in this chapter can go a long way, or even all the way, to relieving and perhaps even curing asthma. But they concentrate mainly on the body. They have some impact on our mental and emotional state but that is not their main purpose. In the case of some asthmatics, however, it is the psychological problems – such as stress for example – which are an important trigger factor, and sometimes one that purely physical therapies can't help. In this situation sufferers may find that the approaches outlined in the following chapter are of more benefit.

CHAPTER 8

Treating your mind and emotions

Therapies for how you think and feel

There is nothing new about asthma nor the link between asthma and emotion. Maimonides, the great physician to the court of the Saracen leader Saladin, commented on the link more than 800 years ago. No-one doubts now that the emotions are involved in the onset of asthma – even though it is rarely the main, or only, cause.

A number of natural therapies are very successful at calming down and even soothing away the sort of mental and emotional strain, or stress, that can aggravate asthma if not trigger it directly. They can be called 'inside-out' therapies in the sense that they work from the inside (your mind and emotions) to the outside (your outer health). Positive thinking, meditation, relaxing the mind through 'visualization' are all inside-out techniques. But first what do we mean by stress exactly? And is it always bad?

The significance of stress

Most of us know what stress is even though it's difficult to define. We are 'in stress' if life becomes a 'trial', if we go around feeling like a kind of pressure cooker, nervous, rigid and 'tight' rather than relaxed and spontaneous as we are supposed to feel. It is a kind of breakdown of the natural free-flowing way the healthy person experiences life. For many people the problem is not the pressure itself but the inability to cope with it satisfactorily – which is why it is sometimes called 'cope-lessness'.

So stress is a convenient word for a combination of both strain and tension, or pressure, and it is particularly significant in asthma because of asthma's known 'psychosomatic' origins and causes. 'Psychosomatic' means basically 'mind and body', so treatments that help the mind are likely also to help the body.

The important thing to remember is that stress is not all bad. Tension is a fact of life. It's part of being human. It may damage some people but it can strengthen others. It is damaging when turned inwards and 'denied' or fought against. The energy – which is what it is – then becomes blocked and misdirected. For example, when people are full of rage and don't express it in any way the actual effort of blocking it may take up much of the energy they could use in a more creative way.

There are two simple rules for making stress work for you rather than against:

- Don't ignore it. Admit it is there; talk about it, write about it - but never ignore it.
- Don't sit and mope. Get up and do something. Go swimming, play music, walk, paint, talk to a friend, do anything – but don't do *nothing*.

Sometimes it helps to get professional help, though, and if you would rather do that there are a number of approaches you may find helpful, ranging from the physical therapies such as yoga and massage mentioned in the previous chapter to more 'psychological' therapies such as counselling and relaxation. In this chapter we'll deal with this last group.

Counselling therapies

As the name suggests, counselling therapies generally encourage you to sit quietly and talk openly about yourself and your problems to a trained and experienced listener, or listeners, who will help you find insights and see solutions for yourself. They include counselling, hypnotherapy and psychotherapy:

- *Counselling* is becoming such a well-organized, regulated and widespread therapy these days it is almost wrong to call it unconventional any longer. Nevertheless it is included because it is very clearly a safe and gentle treatment and extremely important in helping many people cope with major periods of stress and strain, whether a broken marriage, redundancy, debt or sexual difficulties. In Britain and America it is increasingly common to find professional counsellors on the staff of health centres and clinics.

- *Hypnotherapy* (and *Hypnosis*) is a very specific form of psychological treatment, well supported by research, in which trained specialists – and they may be doctors as well as non-medical practitioners – aim to help you deal with unconscious or subconscious mental and emotional distress by placing you into a controlled hypnotic trance and helping you 'get in touch with' the cause or causes of the distress. Once the cause is revealed it may be easier to deal with it consciously through normal counselling or psychotherapy, which is why many hypnotherapists are also psychotherapists. Hypnotherapy can also be a way of learning to relax deeply as well. Some of the relaxation tapes now on the market use a form of very light hypnosis to aid relaxation.

Hypnosis and asthma

Hypnosis has been shown to be effective in asthma in controlled trials. In a study in 1988 at Southampton General Hospital it succeeded in reducing the number of admissions to hospital as well as the amount of drugs administered in the case of 16 patients with chronic asthma. After a year of regular hypnotherapy the number of times the patients had to be admitted to hospital fell from 44 to 13 and the length of time they stayed in fell also. A standard anti-inflammatory drug was able to be withdrawn completely from six of the patients and reduced in eight. None of the patients needed an increase in drug treatment.

- *Psychotherapy*, like counselling, is a method of getting you to understand and face up to psychological problems within yourself by talking them through with a trained listener. *It has nothing to do with psychiatry which is a purely medical discipline based mainly on drug treatment of mental problems.* It can be done on either an individual basis or in a group. There is an enormous variety of psychological therapies available – far more than there is room to list here – and they cover almost every type and style of approach, from the spiritually complex (such as psychosynthesis) to the down-to-earth (such as laughter therapy). Research, particularly in Sweden, is showing that laughter therapy is extremely effective in releasing the sort of tension linked with aggressively repressed, hard-driving 'type A' personality people who may also be prone to asthma.

  Other psychological therapies you are likely to come across are co-counselling (or re-evaluation counselling), encounter therapy, gestalt therapy, psychodrama therapy, bioenergetics, Rogerian therapy, transpersonal psychology and transactional analysis. There are growing numbers of therapists who specialize

STALK and SABRES: How not to die of distress

British cardiologist Dr Peter Nixon believes there is a vital connection between physical effort and psychological break-down, which he has defined as 'the human function curve': when body and mind are required to do more than they can cope with they reach a point of exhaustion, followed by ill-health and finally complete breakdown. He has developed a programme for recovery from 'catastrophic stress' – severe stress leading to a physical breakdown – which he summa-rizes with the colourful acronyms STALK and SABRES. If you are in crisis your first action is to STALK:

STOP everything and take time to re-evaluate what you are doing

THINK through the crisis and try and understand what it means

ACQUIRE information about possible treatment

LEADER: find someone to help you back to health

KNOWLEDGE: know about yourself and your relationship with the world.

Having decided your answers your next step is to perform SABRES:

SLEEP: sleep should be adequate, using hypnotherapy if necessary

AROUSAL should be modulated: do not get too excited or overwrought

BREATHING: avoid over-breathing (hyperventilation)

REST should be balanced out with

EFFORT: gentle to moderate exercise is probably beneficial

SELF-ESTEEM: the recovery of self-esteem through suc-cess.

Dr Nixon, who runs a stress-counselling clinic in London, believes a good therapist should offer support and guidance to people in crisis rather than tell them what to do, and should avoid resort to drugs if at all possible. Ideally, the therapist should be part of a team with different skills who can pool their experience and resources on the patient's behalf.

in 'stress management' (such as Dr Peter Nixon, *see box on page 89*) and often they will be in the best position to guide you towards the right psychological approach if they can't help you themselves.

Relaxation therapies

The very opposite of activity therapies such as dance therapy and 'encounter' therapy, which deal mainly with violent emotion and repressed anger, relaxation therapies aim to encourage a sense of deep inner peace and well-being by getting you to relax to such an extent you enter an almost dream-like state. They require conditions of quiet calm and the minimum of movement. Researchers have found that relaxation training can strongly benefit breathing, particularly in children *(see figure 8)*. The various methods include:

- *Meditation* is popularly seen as sitting in the famous 'lotus' position of the Indian yogis, legs crossed, hands together and eyes closed. But it need not be like this at all. Yoga and meditation are closely linked but it is possible to meditate lying in bed in the morning or sitting on a park bench provided nothing much else is going on around. The important thing is to listen to nothing but your own inner mind, the 'quiet centre' within yourself. 'Silent prayer' can be a form of meditation if you don't actually think but let the thoughts arrive of their own free will. Most of the many formal meditation methods have been imported into the West from the Orient, including the famous Transcendental Meditation (TM) and various yogas like *hatha yoga, raja yoga* and *tantra yoga*.
- *Autogenics* is a sort of Western version of meditation, which combines some of the purposes of meditation with the techniques of auto-suggestion (made famous

MIND/BODY CHANGES

Effect of Tension	Mind/Body Function	Effect of Relaxation
up	Heart rate	down
down	Parasympathetic nervous system	up
up	Blood flow to muscle	down
down	Blood flow to skin	up
down	Blood flow to organs	up
up	Oxygen usage	down
up	Cortisone output	down
down	Food and energy reserves	up
up	Blood pressure	down
up	Muscle tension	down
up	Mental activity (chatter)	down

RESULT
Action

RESULT
Proper function of organs

1. These are general changes. They can be localized to one organ or system.

2. Prolonged tension leads to permanent changes and may lead to disease.

3. Immune mechanisms and antibodies are also affected by tension because of the raised cortisone output.

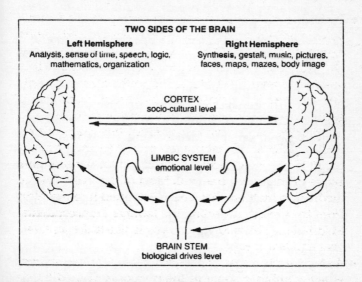

TWO SIDES OF THE BRAIN

Left Hemisphere
Analysis, sense of time, speech, logic, mathematics, organization

Right Hemisphere
Synthesis, gestalt, music, pictures, faces, maps, mazes, body image

CORTEX
socio-cultural level

LIMBIC SYSTEM
emotional level

BRAIN STEM
biological drives level

Fig. 8 The brain hemispheres and stress

by the Frenchman Emile Coué with his *mantra*: 'Every day, in every way, I am getting better and better'). Often called 'passive concentration', it teaches six specific mental exercises to help you (actually your hypothalamus gland) switch off your normal 'fight or flight' responses and 'switch on the rest, relaxation and recreation system'.

- *Visualization* is a method often used in many meditative techniques positively to encourage your mind into a relaxed state by imagining any scene you like that is peaceful and restful. Counting sheep jumping over a fence to get to sleep is exactly the process. Therapeutically it has been used against cancer – patients are encouraged to imagine, for example, good white blood cells gobbling up or destroying harmful red cells – and could be used in the same way in asthma: you could try imagining, for example, your lungs and airways pink with health and full of all the clean, warm air you need.

- *Relaxing tapes and videos* are but the cheapest end of a blossoming market in mechanical aids for relaxation. Tapes and videos, of course, you can listen to or see at any time at home but some health centres offer them as part of a general relaxation programme, such as during 'floating' (floating inside a closed chamber of warm Epsom salts) or 'de-stressing' (lying in a special unit with your head outside, like a personal Turkish bath, so that different temperatures can be applied to your head and body: this apparently fools your mind into relaxing your body!). The British Holistic Medical Association publishes audio-tapes for relaxation as part of its *Tapes for Health* series.

- *Biofeedback* is a way of teaching yourself relaxation (and indeed meditation) by monitoring your relaxation responses with special equipment. For example, you could measure your brain-wave patterns (EEG) or blood pressure while relaxing and, depending on your responses, teach yourself to do more of what works and less of what doesn't. The idea is to help you confirm your mind in the ways it should work for best results for you. One of the most simple and effective tools for the asthmatic is the electrical skin resistance meter (ESR) which indicates arousal and relaxation.

Biofeedback and asthma

A classic study of the effect of biofeedback in helping asthma was carried out as long as 20 years ago at a summer camp in Charleston, West Virginia, where 22 asthmatic children were given deep-muscle relaxation using biofeedback responses. Compared with a group that had no therapy, the asthma in the children who had the biofeedback relaxation improved greatly, as shown by improvements in behaviour rating, peak flow rates, reduction in the number of visits to hospital and in the use of steroid medication. Since then there have been numerous studies of the success of biofeedback in stress reduction.

Summary

It is not always easy, or even possible, to know in advance which of the many 'psychological' therapies is most suitable in any one particular case. One important difference between the different approaches may, however, give you some idea.

Many modern psychotherapies are based on a form of psychology known as 'behaviourist'. According to this theory, everything we do is the result of conditioning and the only way to correct unacceptable behaviour is by 'de-conditioning' or 're-conditioning'. In other words the patient is 're-programmed' into behaviour that conforms to what is normally acceptable through a system of reward and punishment: 'good' behaviour is rewarded and 'bad' behaviour punished. But under this essentially western 'scientific' system the therapist is the one who is deciding what is acceptable behaviour and what is not.

Psychotherapies based largely on Oriental philosophies, on the other hand, are almost the complete opposite: they try to make people aware of their conditioning so that they can discover 'the true self'. The aim of Eastern-style psychotherapies is enlightenment, which is a state of total awareness and 'non-attachment'. Buddhism, for example, and especially Zen Buddhism, teaches this approach through various exercises which usually include meditation – such as the 'movement meditation' known as *zahzen*. Such approaches have a lot to offer the asthmatic, whether physically or psychologically sick.

This may, of course, leave you none the wiser about what will suit you, and work for you. Instead of casting around at random and taking 'pot luck', though, one answer may be what is called 'multi-dimensional treatment'. American therapists Drs Daniel Brown and Erika Fromm, who have studied the mind-body aspects of asthma, favour this sort of multi-disciplinary approach in which a variety of both physical and psychological approaches, conventional and natural, are used together.

Starting with a careful assessment of the patient's condition, identifying among other things the trigger agents, measuring pulmonary functioning and the extent of bronchial activity, assessing the psychological aspects such as the impact of asthma on the patient's behaviour, how the attacks affect his or her self-image, and how relatives and others close to the patient react to his or her attacks, they then devise a programme of treatment.

The treatment recommended by Brown and Fromm includes hypnotism to desensitize the patient against anxiety and panic about the onset of an asthmatic attack, and relaxation and breathing exercises used in a particular technique they have developed known as 'visceral learning'. This helps the patient learn to dilate the bronchial passages and, if the exercises become routine, to stabilize bronchial activity.

The exercises, which consist of 'bellows' and 'expiratory' breathing (see page 78), are combined with visualization. For example, Brown and Fromm ask the patient to imagine he or she is sitting in a comfortable chair with expanding or elastic walls. During an expiratory breathing exercise the patient imagines pushing the walls back with the force of the breath. The patient is helped with peak flow readings that monitor his or her progress. This acts like biofeedback, helping the patient to assess his or her performance from day to day, and reinforcing successful application of breathing techniques when they occur.

CHAPTER 9

Treating your 'subtle body'

How 'energy therapies' can help asthma

'Subtle body' or 'energy' therapies depend for their results on the invisible 'energy fields' that many believe flow through and around the body. So far no-one has been able to measure these fields though practitioners of these therapies, their patients and a number of researchers – such as those at the prestigious Russian Academy of Sciences Institute of Terrestrial Magnetism in Moscow – are convinced they exist because their effects are observable, particularly in the case of such therapies as homoeopathy and acupuncture.

Therapies in this area known to be helpful in cases of asthma are:

- acupuncture
- acupressure
- healing and 'Therapeutic Touch'
- homoeopathy
- reflexology
- shiatsu
- the Metamorphic Technique
- Vacuflex therapy.

Acupuncture

Acupuncture originated thousands of years ago in China apparently when it was discovered that soldiers wounded by arrows sometimes mysteriously recovered from illnesses from which they had been suffering for years. The Chinese started copying the effects using needles (originally made of stone called 'stone piercers') rather than arrows. From those primitive beginnings acupuncture has become today a very precise and delicate art in which needles are used at particular 'acu-points' – there are over 800 of them – along 12 main 'vital energy' (*chi*) pathways called 'meridians'.

In disease, according to the Chinese, the energy flow becomes unbalanced. The acupuncturist can detect this by feeling the pulses at the radial artery of the wrist. The pulses have a variety of different tensions – hardness, fullness, quietness, over- or under-activity – which the skilled acupuncturist can recognize. Various acupoints are connected to different parts of the body and are associated with different conditions, and once the right points are located needles are inserted at varying depths either to stimulate the energy (increase the *yang*, or 'positive energy') or sedate it (increase the *yin*, or negative).

Traditional acupuncture is essentially holistic, treating or 'balancing' the 'energetic harmony' of the person rather than the symptoms of a disease, and so each patient is treated differently. The position of points that might benefit someone varies from patient to patient, and may even change with time. This makes research difficult to carry out but nevertheless acupuncture has proved effective in stopping asthmatic attacks and easing the symptoms.

In one study, in which 19 children with exercise-induced asthma (controlled with oral or aerosol bronchodilators) were treated at both real and sham acupoints, improvements in the symptoms as well as the lung function were reported in the group receiving the real acupuncture whereas those getting the fake acupuncture showed no improvements at all.

Acupressure

Acupressure is another Oriental technique and there is some discussion about which came first: acupressure or acupuncture. The principles of both are identical except acupuncture uses needles and acupressure fingers and thumbs, and sometimes also elbows and knees, to stimulate the body's 'energy points'. You could come across various versions of the technique, including *Do-In*, *Jin Shen*, *Jin Shin*, *Jin Shen Do* and *Shen Tao*, but the most common and well known is *Shiatsu*.

- *Shiatsu* means 'finger pressure' in Japan where the therapy is believed to have originated. As the name implies it is a form of massage therapy in which pressure is applied to various points and areas of the body. Most of the points are the same as used in acupuncture and the technique is often described as 'acupuncture massage'. Both arts share the same philosophy of medicine, their aim being to stimulate the flow of 'energy' (called *ki* in Japanese).

In Japan shiatsu is commonly practised in the home by family members on one another to relieve aches and pain and to restore energy when someone is tired. It is easy enough to do in your own home if you wish although many people prefer to go to a properly-trained specialist. The room where the massage is given should be quiet and simple, with no distractions. The clothes worn should be loose-fitting and made of a natural fabric and the person giving the massage should be absolutely calm and fully responsive to the needs of the person being treated. It is a relaxing form of massage which is of benefit to many asthmatics.

Healing

Healing, better known by most people as 'faith healing' or 'spiritual healing', is probably the simplest, safest and most natural of all methods of healing in that it involves nothing but the touch, or sometimes only the thoughts, of the healer to work. This is not to say that the practice of healing is simply putting your hands on someone and waiting for things to happen. Healers claim that the practice of healing is a 'profound, personal spiritual experience' – as much for the healer as for the person being healed. Working, they say, on physical, mental and emotional levels simultaneously, it is frequently of great power and significance for them both.

Surprising as it may seem, there is actually more research into the therapeutic effects of 'hands-on' healing than any other form of natural therapy, with the exception of hypnotherapy, and that research is continuing. The powers some healers seem to have of alleviating pain and curing disease, even at a distance, is acquiring its own scientific definition. It is now called 'non-local medicine' (from the term 'non-locality' in quantum physics referring to the power of pairs of sub-atomic particles known as *photons* to influence each other over a great distance).

- *Therapeutic Touch*, or 'TT', is a modern version of healing by the laying-on-of-hands. The term is used in countries, particularly the United States, where to call yourself a 'healer' and to claim to heal by, in effect, supernatural means is illegal in many states. Nevertheless TT, now in common use by nurses in clinics and hospitals, is based on the belief in the actual physical transfer of human life energy from the person touching to the person being touched. In other words, where there is tender loving touch there is healing.

There is no mystery about this of course. It happens every day in homes where mothers care for their sick children. The mere act of touching a sick child with love and devotion will have positive results, improving morale and helping fight off illness. But TT does not seem to depend just on faith. There is a growing body of research that show its effects are real.

TT, like other such healing techniques in which the body's own healing powers are reinforced, is available to anyone including asthmatics. It has been shown at least to ease symptoms if not eliminate them altogether and can help to improve the quality of life of any sick person.

Homoeopathy

Homeopathy is a system of medicine first introduced 200 years by a German doctor called Samuel Hahnemann. Based on the principle 'like heals like', homoeopathy claims to heal by the application of minute doses of various substances, from herbs and minerals to sea-shells, linked to the condition to be cured. The doses are usually taken in the form of small tablets.

Because homoeopaths, a bit like Chinese practitioners, see conditions as symptoms of something deeper, and often psychological in origin, there are no 'standard cures' for asthma and self-prescribing is definitely *not* recommended. A responsible homoeopath will insist that each person must have a remedy or combination of remedies based on the homoeopath's careful assessment of the individual. This will include going into someone's background in great detail to gather all possible relevant facts about them and their life so far.

Many conventional doctors don't accept homoeopathic remedies because they say there is no measurable active ingredient in the tablet. Nevertheless homoeopathy has

---

The homoeopathic 'Law of Cure'

Homoeopaths work to the following principles:

- The body has its own self-repairing processes and it's the practitioner's duty to encourage these processes with the minimum of medication.

- The patient must always be treated as a whole, taking all signs and symptoms into consideration.

The body's restorative processes include what are described as 'acute symptoms'. In homoeopathic medicine this means they return if they have been previously suppressed. According to Hering's 'Law of Cure', all cure comes from within out, from the head down, and in the reverse order that the symptoms have appeared in the body. This means – to the alarm of some patients – that symptoms can sometimes become worse before they get better. The more acute and superficial symptoms will be the last to go away if they were the first to appear.

---

an impressive record in a wide range of conditions, including asthma. Most impressive of all, perhaps, it has been shown to work on farm animals as well as pets, both of whom are unlikely to be acting simply to please or because they are in awe of the practitioner (which is what doctors often think causes the results in human patients – the 'placebo effect' referred to earlier).

Homoeopathic remedies have helped cure or alleviate chest conditions, but many homoeopaths insist that homoeopathy cannot be 'mixed' with other techniques and that results only come if pharmaceutical drugs, in particular, are stopped. Nowadays, though, many leading homoeopaths advise asthmatics not to come off their medicines until they are completely better and then only with the consent of their family doctor or hospital consultant. They say that homeopathic remedies *are* compatible with such drugs as *Intal* and *Ventolin*, and it may be that a combination of these approaches allows a gradual

ible with such drugs as *Intal* and *Ventolin*, and it may be that a combination of these approaches allows a gradual reduction of conventional medication. This is the practice at the children's outpatients clinic at the Royal London Homoeopathic Hospital.

The 'London Air Pollution' remedy

Asthmatics often suffer as a result of their working environment. Indoor pollutants such as tobacco smoke, microorganisms in air-conditioned offices, cooling towers, old books and mildewed paper; fibreglass used in insulating material, paint fumes and so on can all trigger an asthma attack (see chapter 2). But homoeopathy claims to be able to desensitize people effectively to many of these substances. British homoeopaths have even produced a 'London Air Pollution' remedy that claims to have helped many asthmatic patients suffering from pollution in Britain's capital.

Reflexology

Reflexology is the science of treating health problems by massaging 'reflex zones' in the feet that are believed to correspond to and link up with different parts of the body. To this extent it has associations with acupuncture and acupressure (see page 98). It is sometimes also called 'reflex zone therapy' or simply 'zone therapy', although 'zone therapists' insist the two are different. By applying pressure to specific reflex points in the feet, usually with the finger and/or thumb, the part of the body affected is believed to be stimulated also. Just as in acupuncture and acupressure, this stimulation is said to promote the body's natural 'balancing' or self-healing mechanism.

One explanation of how reflexology works is that compressing the skin and tissue stimulates the special nerves known as 'sensory receptors' that lie just below the surface of the skin. This stimulation sends its message through the nerves to the spinal cord where it is then dispersed through the central nervous system to produce various effects in connected parts of the body.

The origin of reflexology is uncertain, though it is believed to have come from China to the West. One theory is that in China it may have been a development of acupressure. For example, therapists believe pressure applied to the reflex point on the feet relating to the solar plexus is believed to help the lungs by relaxing the diaphragm and so enabling the lungs to expand more fully and increasing their intake of oxygen.

These days reflexology is practised with considerable success in the West, particularly in Denmark where it is the most frequently used alternative therapy ahead of both acupuncture and homoeopathy. A large number of nurses are trained in reflexology (as they now are in Britain, although not to the official extent they are in Denmark). The success of reflexology, which is practised by trained reflexologists in both private and public companies, in producing a considerable reduction in absenteeism has prompted the Danish government to finance a large-scale research programme in which a number of hospitals and doctors are involved.

The main variations in use are the Metamorphic Technique and Vacuflex therapy:

- *The Metamorphic Technique* A fairly recent development, this sees points on the feet relating to emotional influences which affected you before you were born and which can lead to illnesses later such as asthma. Pressure on the points is believed to remove the stored traumas from those influences and so remove the illnesses themselves.
- *Vacuflex therapy* Vacuflex therapy is a modern 'hi-

tech' version of reflexology. Pressure is applied on all the feet points at once through special felt boots from which the air is withdrawn to create a vacuum. Marks left on the feet are said to indicate which areas of the body need further treatment by special suction pads. This is reminiscent of 'cupping' which is used extensively in Chinese medicine. The special value of the technique is that it is claimed to be more effective than traditional reflexology as well as quicker by covering all the reflexes. Its practitioners claim there is evidence from case studies of benefit in cases of both asthma and allergies generally although there is, as yet, no scientific research to back this up.

Summary

By dealing with all levels of dis-ease – mental and emotional as well as physical – the subtle energy therapies seem to be particularly well suited to the needs of a condition such as asthma and so well worth a try. Almost all natural therapies take time to work – there are few 'quick fixes' such as conventional medicine tries to offer – so don't expect miracles. Patience and a certain amount of effort on your part is usually required to achieve the full benefit, but if you are prepared for this there is a chance of good results.

Certainly there seems to be evidence the therapies mentioned in these pages are likely to be able to help in a large number of cases – though, as said before, finding and choosing the right therapist is important. In the final chapter we'll look at various ways of doing this.

CHAPTER 10

How to find and choose a natural therapist

Tips and guidelines for seeking out reliable help

It is unfortunately not as easy as it should be to find the right therapist. Although natural medicine is enjoying a boom and everyone seems to want to make use of it, diversity, competition between groups and duplication within therapies has made the task a difficult one in most countries in which they are rising in popularity. It is the main purpose of *The Natural Way With* series to help you find the right gentle therapy for your condition – but finding the right practitioner or therapist is in some ways the harder task.

The best solution is almost always personal recommendation, and this applies as much to doctors as non-medical practitioners. Go to someone a friend or someone you trust has recommended. As a rule of thumb it cannot be bettered. But if you still cannot find a good recommendation what next? There are several options:

● Go to your local doctor's clinic or health centre and ask their advice. It may take some courage and you may not get a sympathetic response. But it is worth a try, and you may get a pleasant surprise. You may find they have the very person you need – either someone who helps at the clinic or someone to whom patients are referred (which means, in countries with a state health service, possibly free treatment).

- Your nearest natural health centre may be able to help, or even a natural health practitioner whom you know is not the right person for you but who may be prepared to recommend someone else. This way is not as good as personal recommendation but therapists who specialize in natural therapy tend to know who else is at work in their area and, more importantly, who is any good. You can find the names of centres and individual practitioners to approach from healthfood shops, *Yellow Pages* or local listings in newspapers, magazines, citizen advice and information centres and libraries. If you are involved with computers and have a modem make use of computer network lists. A particularly good place to investigate is any natural health centre in your area with several practitioners all with different skills. The better centres have a system where a patient contacting them for help can be offered a consultation in which his or her case is considered by a panel of practitioners and then a method of treatment and a therapist or therapists recommended. Such an approach is still in its infancy, though, so it may be hard to find.
- Failing a local recommendation or the availability of an enlightened group practice, the next step is to contact any of the national therapy 'umbrella' organizations and ask for their list(s) of registered organizations or practitioners. Their addresses are listed in Appendix A. They may charge for their lists (especially for postage and packing) and insist you select not only which therapy but also, because there is still no one recognized organization for each therapy in many countries, which particular organization you want a members' list of. If you can afford it ask for all of them.

---

10 ways of finding a therapist

- word-of-mouth (usually the best method)
- your local family medical centres
- your local natural health centres
- your local healthfood shops
- health farms and beauty treatment centres
- local patient support groups
- national therapy organizations (but see below)
- computer networks (you need a 'modem')
- public libraries and information centres
- local *Yellow Pages*, newspapers and magazines.

Checking professional organizations

Whether or not you have found a therapist straight away it is still a good idea to check on their professional background. This becomes almost essential if you are picking a name from a list rather than following a recommendation from a friend. Just because a therapist belongs to an organization doesn't mean he or she comes with a guarantee. Some organizations do no more vetting of their members than making sure they've paid their membership fees.

The first thing to do is to check the status of the individual associations or professional organizations whose names you have got. A good association will publish the information clearly and simply in the same booklet as its members' list. Few seem to, however, and so you may have to ring them up or write to them. The following are the sort of questions you should try and get answered:

- When was the association founded? (Groups spring up all the time and you may find it useful to know if they have been going 50 years or started yesterday.)
- How many members does it have? (Size will give you a good idea of its public acceptance and genuine aims.)

- Is it a charity or educational trust – with a formal constitution, an elected committee and published accounts – or is it a private limited company? (Private companies can be secretive and self-serving.)
- Is it part of a larger network of professional organizations? (Groups that go their own way are on balance more suspect than those who 'join in'.)
- Does the association have a code of ethics, complaints mechanism and disciplinary procedures? If so, what are they?
- Is the association linked to one particular school or college? (One that is may have no independent assessment of its membership; the head of the association may also be head of the college.)
- What are the criteria for membership? (If it is graduation from one particular school or college the same problem arises as above.)
- Are members covered by professional indemnity insurance against accident and malpractice?

Checking training and qualifications

Next you may want to try and satisfy yourself about their training and qualifications. A good listing will, again, describe the qualifications and say what the initials after every member's name mean. Yet again, few seem to. So it's a case of ringing or writing to find out. Questions to ask are the following:

- How long is the training?
- Is it full-time or part-time?
- Does it include seeing patients under supervision?
- Is the qualification recognized?
- If so, by whom?

The British Medical Association's opinon

In its long-awaited second report into the practice of natural medicine in Britain, published in June 1993, the British Medical Association recommended that anyone seeking the help of what is called a 'non-conventional therapist' – doctor or patient – should ask the following questions:

- Is the therapist registered with a professional organization?
- Does the professional organization have
  a public register?
  a code of practice?
  an effective disciplinary procedure and sanction?
  a complaints mechanism?
- What qualification does the therapist hold?
- What training was involved in getting the qualification(s)?
- How many years has the therapist been practising?
- Is the therapist covered by professional indemnity insurance?

The BMA said that although it would like to see natural therapies regulated by law, with a single regulating body for each therapy, it did not think that all therapies needed regulating. For the majority, it said, 'the adoption of a code of practice, training structures and voluntary registration would be sufficient.'

Complementary Medicine: New Approaches to Good Practice (Oxford University Press, 1993).

Making the choice

The final choice is a matter of using a combination of common sense and intuition and giving someone a try. But do not hesitate to double-check with them when you see them that the information in the listing agrees with what they tell you – nor to cancel an appointment (give at least 24 hours notice if you can) or to walk out if you do not like anything about the person, the place or the treatment. The important advice at all times is to ask questions, as many as you need to, and use your intuition. Never forget: it is your body and mind!

What is seeing a natural therapist like?

It a word, different. But it is also very natural. Since most therapists, even in those countries with state health systems, still work mainly privately there is no established uniform or common outlook. Though they may all share more or less a belief in the principles outlined in chapter 7 you are liable to come across individuals as different as chalk from cheese, representing all walks of life, from the rich to the poor, the politically left to the politically right. That means you will come across as much variety in dress, thinking and behaviour as there are fashions, from the elegant and formal to the positively informal and 'woolly-haired' (though, for image reasons, many now wear a white coat to look more like a doctor!).

Equally, you will find their premises very different – reflecting their attitudes to their work and the world. Some will present a 'brass plaque' image, working in a clinic or room away from home with receptionist and brisk efficiency, while others will see you in their living room surrounded by pot plants and domestic clutter. Remember, though, image may be some indication of status but it is little guarantee of ability. You are as likely to find a therapist of quality working from home as one in a formal clinic.

There are some characteristics, however, probably the most important ones, you will find common to all natural therapists. They will:

- give you far more time than you are used to with a family doctor. An initial consultation will rarely last less than an hour, and often longer. During it they will ask you all about yourself so they can form a proper understanding of what makes you tick and what may be the fundamental cause(s) of your problem

- charge you for their time and for any remedies they prescribe, which they may well sell you themselves from their own stocks. But many therapists offer reduced fees, and even waive fees altogether, for deserving cases or for people who genuinely cannot afford it.

Sensible precautions

- Though most practitioners practise for fees no ethical person will ask for fees in advance of treatment unless for special tests or medicines, but even this is unusual. If you are asked for a deposit of any sort ask exactly what for and if you don't like the reasons don't pay.
- Be sceptical of anyone who 'guarantees' you a cure. No-one (not even doctors) can.
- Be very wary of stopping drugs prescribed by your family doctor on the therapist's insistence without first talking things over with your doctor. Non-medical therapists know little about pharmaceutical drugs and there may be danger to yourself if you stop suddenly or without preparation.
- If you are female feel free to have someone with you if you need to undress and if being accompanied makes you feel more comfortable. No ethical therapist will refuse such a request, and if they do have nothing more to do with them.

What to do if things go wrong

The most important thing to decide is whether you think the therapist has done his or her absolute best to get you better without hurting or harming you in any way.

Failure to cure you is not an offence (the truth is it is probably as much a disappointment to the therapist as it is to you) but failure to take proper care and treat you with professional respect is. If this should happen to you, and you feel it is as the result of behaviour which you regard as either incompetent or unethical, you could consider the following actions:

- If you feel the therapist was doing his or her best to help – and most obviously try to – but simply wasn't good enough it might be as well, for the safety of future patients as much as for the therapist's sake, to talk the problem over with him or her first. The therapist may be oblivious of his or her shortcomings and be not only grateful for your constructive honesty but also see a way to make amends and help you further. But if the situation is more serious than this then you have no option but either to turn your back on the whole episode or take action. If you decide to take further action the courses open to you are:
- Report the therapist to their professional association or society if they have one. (Don't expect this to lead to dramatic changes however. Because unconventional medicine still belongs in many ways to an unestablished, and even sometimes anti-establishment, subculture – it has been called 'the folk medicine of the masses' – it exists in many countries still in a sort of unregulated limbo world in which pretty well anything goes and there are few official controls. This can have its advantages of course: the better and more original practitioners can experiment and change direction at will in a way they wouldn't be allowed to do if they were tied up in rules and regulations as doctors are. But it also means there is little or no professional comeback if they don't behave in a way you like or think they should. Even if they belong to a profes-

sional organization – and, in Britain at least, no practitioner who is not medically trained has to belong to any organization – those organizations have little or no real power to do anything to a member who breaks the rules. In Britain if they expel someone that person is still free to practise under exiting common law provided they don't break any civil or criminal law.)

- Tell anyone and everyone you come across about your experience, especially the person who recommended the therapist if this applies, and tell the therapist you are doing so (but make sure you are telling the truth: deliberately spreading lies that damage someone's reputation and livelihood is a criminal offence). Practitioners who get themselves a bad reputation are quickly out of business – and rightly so – and to that extent, at least, they are under pressure to behave professionally, and they know it. Ultimately that is your only guarantee. But it is also the best guarantee.

- In the very worst case, which is always possible though rare, you can resort to the civil or criminal law – that is, you can sue or bring a charge for assault – either through a lawyer or by going direct to the police. Alternatively citizens' rights or advice bureaux may be able to help.

Summary

The reality is that although the opportunity is there, resulting in the occasional tabloid newspaper headline, there are few real crooks or charlatans in natural therapy. Despite the myth, there is little real money in it unless the therapist is very busy – and if he or she is the chances are high it is because he or she is good. In fact you are just as likely to find bad practitioners in orthodox medicine and among the ranks of the so-called 'qualified' as among those who work quietly alone at

home with no formal training at all. No-one can know **everything** and no-one qualified in anything, including **medicine**, has to get 100 per cent in their exams to be **able** to practise. Perfection is an ideal not a reality and to **err** is human.

It is very much for this reason that taking control of your own health is perhaps the single most important lesson underlying the series of books of which this is part. For taking control means taking responsibility for the choices you make, and taking responsibility for choices we now know to be one of the most significant factors in successful treatment, whether of yourself or through the intermediate services of a therapist. No-one else but you can decide on a practitioner and no-one else but you should decide also if that practitioner is any good or not, whether they are a conventional doctor or a natural therapist, or both. You will know very easily, and probably very quickly, if they are any good by the way you feel about them and their therapy and by whether or not you get any better.

If you are not happy about them or your progress the decision is yours whether to stay or move on – and continue moving until you find the right therapist for you. But do not despair if you don't find the right person first time, and above all never give up hope. There is almost bound to be the right person for you somewhere and your determination to get well is the best resource you have for finding them.

Above all, bear in mind that many people before you who have taken this route have not only been helped beyond their most optimistic dreams but have also found a close and trusted helper who they, and their family, can turn to in times of trouble – and who may even become a friend for life.

APPENDIX A

Useful organizations

The following listing of organizations is for information only and does not imply any endorsement, nor do the organizations listed necessarily agree with the views expressed in this book.

INTERNATIONAL

International Federation of Practitioners of Natural Therapeutics
46 Pulens Crescent
Sheet
Petersfield
Hampshire GU31 4DH, UK.
Tel 0730 266790
Fax 0730 260058

AUSTRALASIA

Association of Asthma Foundations of Australia
Unit 3
46 Geils Court
Deakin
ACT 2600, Australia.

Asthma Foundation of New Zealand
PO Box 1459
Wellington, New Zealand.

Australian Natural Therapists Association
PO Box 308
Melrose Park
South Australia 5039.
Tel 8297 9533
Fax 8297 0003

Australian Traditional Medicine Society
PO Box 442 *or*
Suite 3, First Floor
120 Blaxland Road
Ryde
New South Wales 2112
Australia.
Tel 2808 2825
Fax 2809 7570

New Zealand Natural Health Practitioners Accreditation Board
PO Box 37-491
Auckland, New Zealand.
Tel 9 625 9966
Supported by 15 therapy organizations.

NORTH AMERICA

Allergy Information Association
25 Poynter Drive, Suite 7
Weston
Ontario, Canada.
Tel 718 624 6495

American Academy of Medical Preventics
6151 West Century Boulevard
Suite 1114
Los Angeles
California 90045, USA.
Tel 213 645 5350

American Association of Naturopathic Physicians
2800 East Madison Street
Suite 200
Seattle
Washington 98112, USA

or

PO Box 20386
Seattle
Washington 98102, USA.
Tel 206 323 7610
Fax 206 323 7612

American Holistic Medical Association
6728 Old McLean Village Drive
McLean, VA 22101, USA
Tel 703 556 9222

Association for the Care of Asthma (ACA)
233 S 10th Street Sta 550
Blumic Life Science Building
Philadelphia
Pennsylvania 19107-5541, USA.
Tel 215 955 8912.

Asthma & Allergy Foundation of America (AAFA)
1125 15th Street, NW Sta 502
Washington DC 20005, USA.
Tel 202 466 7643.

Canadian Holistic Medical Association
700 Bay Street
PO Box 101, Suite 604
Toronto
Ontario M5G 1Z6, Canada.
Tel 416 599 0447

National Allergy and Asthma Network
3554 Chain Bridge Road, Ste 200
Fairfax
Vermont 22030-2709, USA.
Tel 703 385 4403.

National Foundation for Asthma
PO Box 50304
Tucson
Arizona 85703, USA.

Solgar Nutritional Research Center
Ocean Pines
11017 Manklin Meadows Lane
Berlin
Maryland 21811, USA.
Tel 410 641 7411

SOUTHERN AFRICA

Food Allergy and Intolerance Society
PO Box 22184
Glenashley 4022
South Africa.

South African Homoeopaths, Chiropractors & Allied Professions Board
PO Box 17055
Groenkloof 0027
South Africa.
Tel 2712 466 455

UK & EIRE

Asthma Society of Ireland
24 Anglesea Street
Dublin 2, Eire.
Tel 010 3531 671 6551

British Allergy Foundation
St Bartholomews Hospital
West Smithfield
London EC1A 7BE.
Tel 071-600 6127

British Complementary Medicine Association
St Charles Hospital
Exmoor Street
London W10 6DZ.
Tel 081-964 1205
Fax 081-964 1207

British Holistic Medical Association
179 Gloucester Place
London NW1 6DX.
Tel 071-262 5299

British Homoeopathic Association
27a Devonshire Street
London W1N 1RJ.
Tel 071-935 2163.
Promotes homoeopathy by medically-qualified practitioners only. Linked to the Faculty of Homoeopathy at the Royal London Homoeopathic Hospital and supplies a register.

British Lung Foundation
18 Peterborough Mews
London SW6 3BL.
Tel 071-371 7704.

British Medical Acupuncture Society
Newton House
Newton Lane
Lower Whitley
Warrington
Cheshire WA4 4JA.
Tel 0925-730727.
Membership limited to doctors, dentists and vets trained in acupuncture.

British Society for Allergy and Clinical Immunology
55 New Cavendish Street
London W1M 7RE.
Tel 071-486 0531.

British Thoracic Society
1 St Andrews Place
London NW1 4LB.
Tel 071-486 7766.

**Council for Complementary &
Alternative Medicine**
179 Gloucester Place
London NW1 6DX.
Tel 071-724 9103
Fax 071-724 5330

**Institute for Complementary
Medicine**
PO Box 194
London SE16 1QZ.
Tel 071-237 5165
Fax 071-237 5175

National Asthma Campaign
Providence House
Providence Place
London N1 0NT.
Tel 071-226 2260.
Helpline 0345 010203
(9am-9pm Mon-Fri, local rate).

**Society of Teachers of the
Alexander Technique (STAT)**
20 London House
266 Fulham Road
London SW10 9EL
Tel 071-351 0828

Yoga for Health Foundation
Ickwell Bury
Biggleswade
Bedfordshire SG18 9EF.
Tel 076-727 271

APPENDIX B

Useful further reading

An A-Z of Alternative Medicine, Brent Hafen and Kathryn Frandson (Sheldon Press, UK, 1984)

Asthma Action Plan: Alternative Ways to Treat Asthma, John Chapman (Thorsons, UK, 1991)

Asthma - Who cares? (The Asthma Training Centre, Stratford-on-Avon, Warwickshire, UK, 1993)

Coping Successfully with Your Child's Asthma, Paul Carson (Sheldon Press, UK, 1987)

Diets to Help Hay Fever and Asthma, Roger Newman Turner (Thorsons, UK, 1989)

Eating and Allergies, Robert Eagle (Futura, UK, 1982)

E for Additives, Maurice Hanssen (Thorsons, UK, 1987)

Hypnosis and Behavioral Medicine, Daniel Brown and Erika Fromm (New Jersey, USA, 1987)

Naturopathic Medicine, Roger Newman Turner (Thorsons, UK, 1984)

Mind-Body Medicine: How to Use Your Mind for Better Health, ed Daniel Goleman and Joel Gurin (Consumer Reports Books, USA, 1993)

Stress Master, Richard Terry Lovelace (John Wiley, UK, 1990)

The Essential Book of Herbal Medicine, Simon Mills (Arkana, UK, 1991)

The Family Guide to Homoeopathy, Andrew Lockie (Hamish Hamilton, UK, 1990)

Viruses, Allergies and the Immune System, Jan de Vries (Mainstream Publishing, UK, 1989)

Index